M.P. Merlini R.J.A.M. van Dongen M. Dusmet (Eds.)

Surgery of the Deep Femoral Artery

With 76 Figures

Springer-Verlag
Berlin Heidelberg New York London Paris
Tokyo Hong Kong Barcelona Budapest

PD Dr. med. MARCO P. MERLINI
Department of Surgery
Hopital, La Chaux-de-Fonds
Rue de Chasseral 20
CH-2300 La Chaux-de-Fonds
Switzerland

Prof. Dr. med. Dr. h.c. R.J.A.M. VAN DONGEN
P.C. Hoffstraat 153-hs
NL-1071 BT Amsterdam
The Netherlands

Dr. med. MICHAEL DUSMET
Department of Surgery
Centre Hospitalier Universitaire Vaudois
CH-1011 Lausanne
Switzerland

Cover photograph: Anatomic plate (RL 12624) (ca 1501) by Leonardo da Vinci (1452–1519), reproduced by permission of The Royal Collection, Her Majesty Queen Elizabeth II.

ISBN 3-540-58067-0 Springer-Verlag Berlin Heidelberg New York
ISBN 0-387-58067-0 Springer-Verlag New York Berlin Heidelberg

Library of Congress Cataloging-in-Publication Data. Surgery of the Deep Femoral Artery / Marco P. Merlini, (ed.). p. cm. ISBN 3-540-58067-0 (alk. paper). — ISBN 0-387-58067-0 (alk. paper) 1. Femoral artery—Surgery. I. Merlini, Marco P. [DNLM: 1. Femoral Artery—surgery. WG 595.F3 S961 1994] RD550.S87 1994 617.5′82—cd20 DNLM/DLC for Library of Congress 94-12558

Printed in Germany

Cover design: Struve & Partner, Heidelberg
Typesetting: Best-set Typesetter Ltd., Hong Kong
24/3130-5 4 3 2 1 0 – Printed on acid-free paper

To Maximilien, Nicolas
and Jessica

Foreword

Circulation through the deep femoral artery and its branches is critical to patients with aortoiliac and infrainguinal arteriosclerosis. It is, accordingly, essential that all physicians who are seriously interested in treating patients with lower extremity ischemia have a good working knowledge of this crucial artery's anatomy and function. It is equally essential that they be aware of arteriosclerotic disease patterns that involve this important artery, how these patterns can be accurately defined, and, most importantly, what therapeutic options are available and when they should be used.

All this important information relating to the deep femoral artery and its surgical significance is included in Dr. Merlini's fine volume. Eighteen authors have contributed 11 well-edited and nicely illustrated chapters that provide all the facts that the committed vascular surgeon would ever want to know about the deep femoral artery and how it should be managed in patients with lower limb ischemia. Although some of the chapters overlap in some areas, this adds to the value of the book since the different authors are all acknowledged experts and their varying perspectives are beneficial to a reader seeking to formulate his own unbiased views.

Dr. Merlini and his collaborators have succeeded in putting together a book which will be valuable to all those who treat lower extremity arteriosclerotic ischemia. It is worthwhile for all vascular surgeons to read this volume since it provides important and relevant background information on this topic. This book will also serve as a reference source of factual information and appropriate literature citations for both trainees and seasoned surgeons seeking to know more about the deep femoral artery and its role in the treatment of lower extremity ischemia. It is certain to become a frequently used and often quoted addition to any vascular surgery library.

Frank J. Veith, MD, FACS
Chief of Vascular Surgical Services,
Montefiore Medical Center, and
Professor of Surgery,
Albert Einstein College of Medicine
New York

Preface

. . . . you will need to acquire a complete knowledge of the veins and arteries . . . .
(Leonardo da Vinci)

The deep femoral is the main artery to the thigh and the main collateral vessel of the lower limb. Intended for a specific vascular bed, it has, like other arteries, the biological particularity of extending its function to a much larger area. Ensuring the vascularization of the osteoarticular and muscular structures of the thigh, it allows us to stand, walk, jump, and run. As a collateral vessel, it can compensate completely for a superficial femoral artery obstruction and maintain the function and the trophicity of the lower limb.

Little is known about the hemodynamics of the deep femoral artery, yet its potentialities are remarkable, going far beyond that which can be done by a thigh bypass in case of an occlusion of the superficial femoral artery. It has actually been known for a long time that the blood flow through an undiseased deep femoral artery is twice the flow through a femoropopliteal bypass. The deep femoral artery also establishes the link between the collateral vessels of the trunk and those of the lower limb and contributes towards compensating for an obstruction of the iliac axes. In this situation, it constitutes the reentry route into the lower limb for the collateral parietal and visceral systems coming from the aorta. It is truly the central segment of a complex network parallel to the main vascular axis.

Arteriosclerosis and occasionally a trauma can affect the deep femoral artery. Such lesions, possibly associated with a proximal obstructive disease, of the superficial femoral or crural arteries, can mean the loss of the leg, of physical integrity, and of the freedom to move about and can lead to suffering for the individual. Thus, maintaining or reestablishing its blood flow is often the goal of the vascular surgeon involved in limb salvage.

This book describes this artery in a normal situation and in the event of superficial femoral obstruction. In the latter case, its role cannot be dissociated from the condition of the aortoiliac and crural circulation. The techniques devised and developed to restore the deep femoral flow are presented from this perspective. Knowing them makes it possible on many an occasion to avoid a major amputation by performing a nontraumatizing procedure.

I sincerely thank Miss Corinne Scheidegger for her perfect organizational work which made it possible to publish this book.

February 1994 MARCO P. MERLINI

Contents

List of Contributors

Victor M. Bernhard, MD, FACS
Professor of Surgery and Chairman
Vascular Surgery Section
College of Medicine, University of Arizona
Tucson, Arizona
USA

William L. Breckwoldt, MD
Assistant Clinical Professor of Surgery
Tufts University School of Medicine
Boston, Massachusetts
USA

Gene L. Colborn, PhD
Professor of Anatomy
Director of the Center of Clinical Anatomy
Medical College of Georgia
Atlanta, Georgia
USA

Thomas F. Dodson, MD, FACS
Assistant Professor of Surgery
Emory University School of Medicine
Atlanta, Georgia
USA

René J.A.M. van Dongen, MD
Prof. Dr. med., Dr. h.c., FACA, FICA
Emeritus Ordinarius of the University of Amsterdam
Head of the Department of Vascular Surgery
Boerhaave Kliniek
Amsterdam
The Netherlands

Michael Dusmet, MD
Chief Resident
Department of Surgery
Centre Hospitalier Universitaire Vaudois
Lausanne
Switzerland

Stephen W. Gray, PhD
Professor Emeritus of Anatomy
Associate Director of the Thalia and Michael Carlos Center for Surgical Anatomy and Technique
Emory University School of Medicine
Consultant to the Medical Staff for Congenital Anomalies
The Piedmont Hospital
Atlanta, Georgia
USA

Edward V. Kinney, MD
4001 Kresge Way
Suite 220
Louisville, Kentucky
USA

Brian Lange, MD
Staff Vascular Surgeon
801 Broadway
Seattle, Washington
USA

Alan B. Lumsden, MBChB
Alfred and Adelle Davis Distinguished Fellow in Surgical Anatomy and Technique
Fellow in Vascular Surgery
Emory University School of Medicine
Atlanta, Georgia
USA

Marco P. Merlini, MD, FRSM, FACA, FCCP, FICS
Privat-Docent and Agrégé at the Faculty of Medicine Lausanne
Switzerland
Head of the Department of Surgery
Hôpital, La Chaux-de-Fonds
Switzerland
Médecin-Adjoint of the Department of Surgery
Centre Hospitalier Universitaire Vaudois
Lausanne
Switzerland

Thomas F. O'Donnell Jr., MD, FACS
Chairman (pro tempore)
Department of Surgery
Tufts University School of Medicine
Chief of Surgery and Chief of Vascular Surgery
New England Medical Center
Boston, Massachusetts
USA

Alfred V. Persson, MD
Medical Director
The Vascular Lab, Metrowest Medical Center
Framingham, Massachusetts
USA

John E. Skandalakis, MD, PhD, FACS
Chris Carlos Distinguished Professor of Surgical Anatomy and Technique
Director of the Thalia and Michael Carlos Center for Surgical Anatomy and Technique and the Alfred A. Davis Research Center for Surgical Anatomy and Technique
Emory University School of Medicine
Senior Attending Surgeon
The Piedmont Hospital
Clinical Professor of Surgery
Medical College of Georgia
Atlanta, Georgia
USA

Lee J. Skandalakis, MD
Alfred and Adelle Davis Distinguished Fellow in Surgical Anatomy and Technique
Emory University School of Medicine
Attending Surgeon

The Piedmont Hospital
Atlanta, Georgia
USA

Michel Y. Suter, MD
Chief Resident
Department of Surgery
Centre Hospitalier Universitaire Vaudois
Lausanne
Switzerland

Jonathan B. Towne, MD, FACS
Professor and Chairman
Vascular Surgery
Medical College of Wisconsin
Milwaukee, Wisconsin
USA

Frits Vaas, MD
Former Head of the Surgical Department of the Lievensberg Hospital
Bergen op Zoom
The Netherlands

1 Surgical Anatomy of the Deep Femoral Artery

A.B. Lumsden, G.L. Colborn, L.J. Skandalakis,
T.F. Dodson, S.W. Gray, and J.E. Skandalakis

I'll do what Mead and Cheselden advise, to keep those limbs and preserve those eyes (Alexander Pope)

John Basmajian (1971) in *Method of Anatomy* referred to the deep femoral artery (DFA) as "no mean vessel." Its clinical importance has been emphasized subsequently by numerous authors (Morris et al. 1961; Leeds and Gilfillan 1961; Martin et al. 1972). We owe our modern anatomical and clinical knowledge of the DFA to the vascular surgeon (Chleborad and Dawson 1990; Hershey and Auer 1974; Martin and Jamieson 1974), the radiologist (Beales et al. 1971), the surgical physiologist, and, of course, the gross human anatomist, a rare and rapidly vanishing phenomenon of our times (Shoeffer 1942; Hollinshead 1969; Cunningham 1981; Skandalakis and Gray 1969, 1983; Skandalakis et al. 1974; Skandalakis 1980, 1984).

The DFA is a relatively small, but dynamic artery, providing a vascular bridge from the pelvic vessels to the vessels around the knee and lower leg. Martin (1972) said of this vessel: "... the anatomy of the profunda is such that there are excellent anastomoses above in the cruciate anastomosis and below with the recurrent tibial vessels." This rich collateral pathway may provide adequate distal perfusion even with complete occlusion of the superficial femoral artery (SFA). Under these conditions it is the main arterial conduit of the leg (Waibel and Wolff 1966).

Surgical Anatomy of the Deep Femoral Artery

The common femoral artery (CFA) begins at the inguinal ligament as a continuation of the external iliac artery (EIA) and divides 3–5 cm (Fig. 1) below the ligament (Leeds and Gilfillan 1961) into the DFA and SFA. A reduction in caliber of the CFA at its bifurcation serves as a guide to the origin of the concealed DFA. The SFA continues through the femoral triangle, enters the subsartorial canal, and ends at the adductor opening in the adductor magnus muscle, where it continues as the popliteal artery (PA).

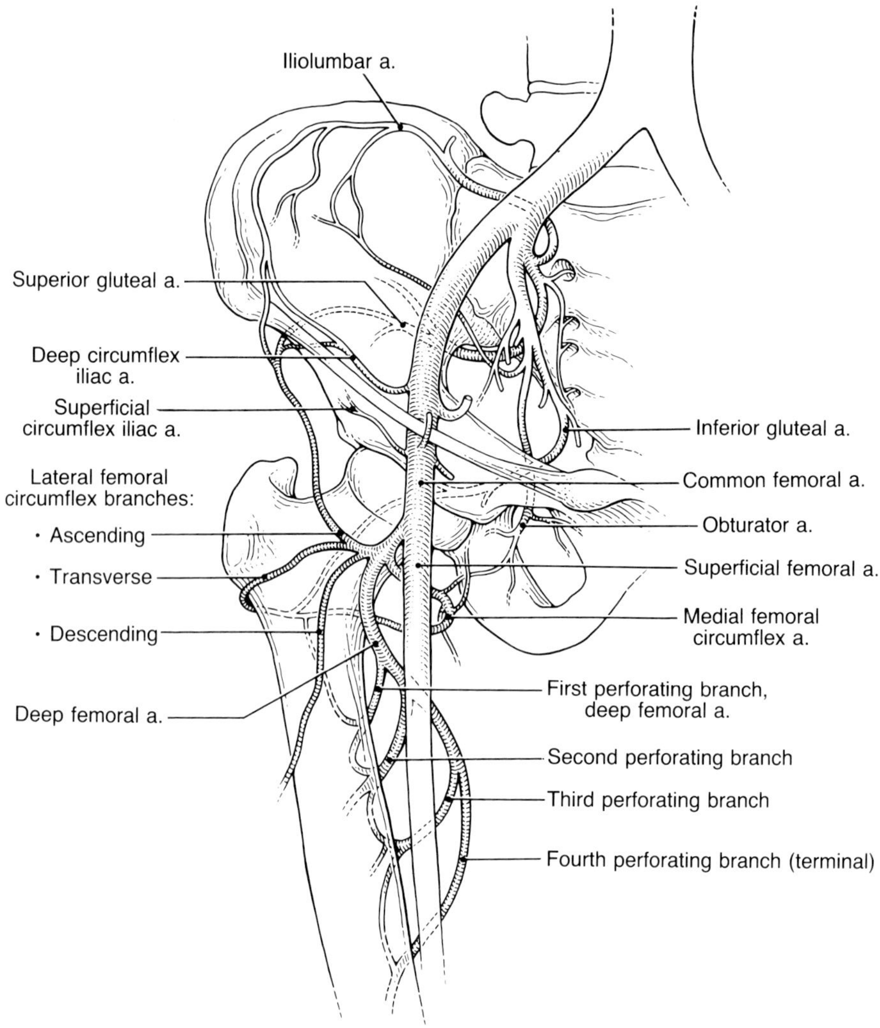

Fig. 1. The origin of the deep femoral artery (DFA) from the common femoral artery (CFA) 3.5–5.0 cm below the inguinal ligament. The rich anastomosis around the femoral head and with the pelvic vessels is evident

There are several important variations in the origin of the DFA (Vaas 1975). The level of origin is variable. In 50% of cases it arises 3.5–5.0 cm below the inguinal ligament. However, in 25% of cases it is 5.0–8.5 cm distal to the ligament, and in the remaining 25% it may originate behind or even above the inguinal ligament (Gray 1985; Haimovici 1984).

At its origin the DFA arises from the posterolateral aspect of the CFA in 40% of cases. However, it may be posterior (37%),

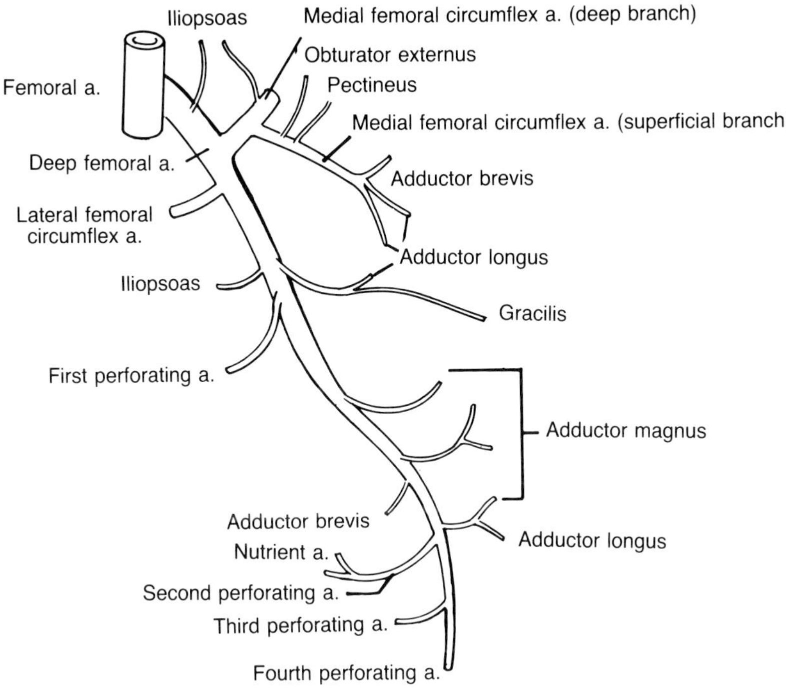

Fig. 2. The deep femoral artery (DFA) has numerous branches through which it supplies most of the thigh musculature and a nutrient artery to the femur

lateral (12%), posteromedial (9%), or, in rare situations, arise from the medial aspect (2%) (Martin et al. 1968). Its caliber is smaller than the SFA (Martin et al. 1968). Siddharth et al. (1985) reported the diameter to range from 4 to 9 mm (median, 5.5 mm).

Via its many branches the DFA supplies most of the thigh musculature and provides articular branches to the hip and knee joints. It is also the nutrient artery to the femur and forms a collateral circulation which links the iliac system of the pelvis proximally to the popliteal vessels at the knee (Fig. 2).

The artery is approximately 30 cm long and may be conveniently described as occurring in three parts: (1) the proximal part measures 12.5 cm, begins at the CFA, and lies in the groove between the psoas and pectineus. It then crosses anterior to the pectineus, behind the adductor longus, where it is sandwiched between the longus anteriorly and the brevis posteriorly; (2) the intermediate part, 5 cm long, lies posterior to the vastus medialis, covered by the thin translucent fascia of the muscle; (3) a 12.5-cm distal or asperal part is adjacent to the linea aspera of the femur, bridged by the insertions of adductor magnus.

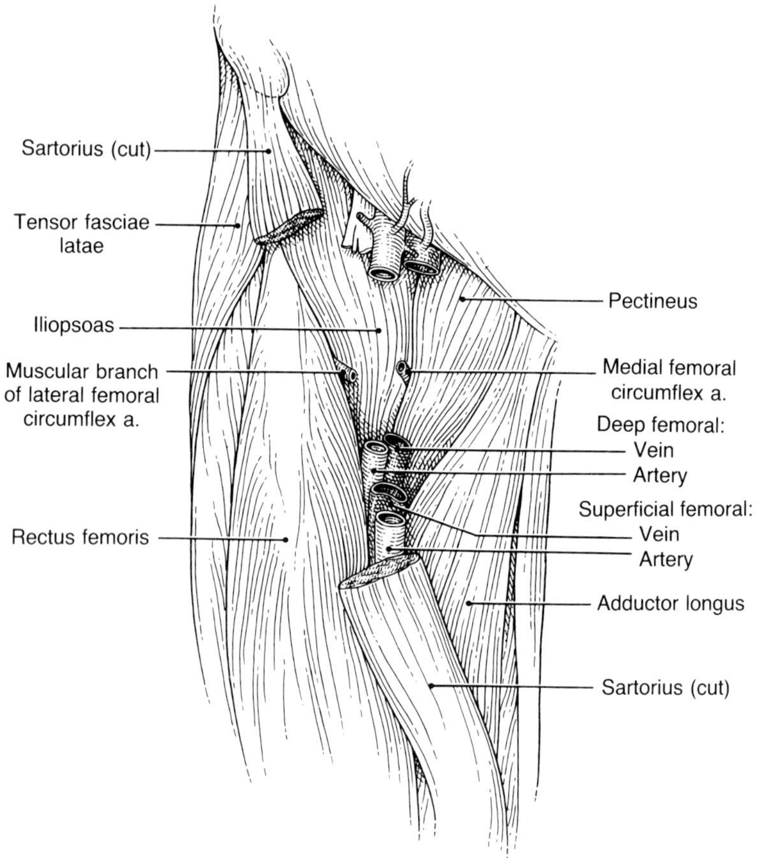

Fig. 3. At the apex of the femoral triangle, the deep femoral vessels lie directly posterior to the superficial femoral vessels. The lateral circumflex artery can be seen passing out of the femoral triangle under cover of the sartorius muscle (cut away), while the medial circumflex passes deeply between the psoas and the pectineus. (Modified from Anderson 1991)

From its origin the DFA winds inferiorly in a loose half spiral. It initially curves posterolaterally away from the CFA and passes deeply out of the femoral triangle between pectineus and adductor longus muscle. As it descends it lies sequentially on the iliopsoas, pectineus, adductor brevis, and adductor magnus muscles. Descending posterior to the adductor longus, it continues its gentle arc such that it subsequently crosses from lateral to medial deep to the SFA and femoral vein. Other variations in the course of the DFA have been noted. Schrutz (1894) reported it passing medially in front of the SFA and vein, while Johnson (1912) reported the DFA passing laterally in front of the SFA.

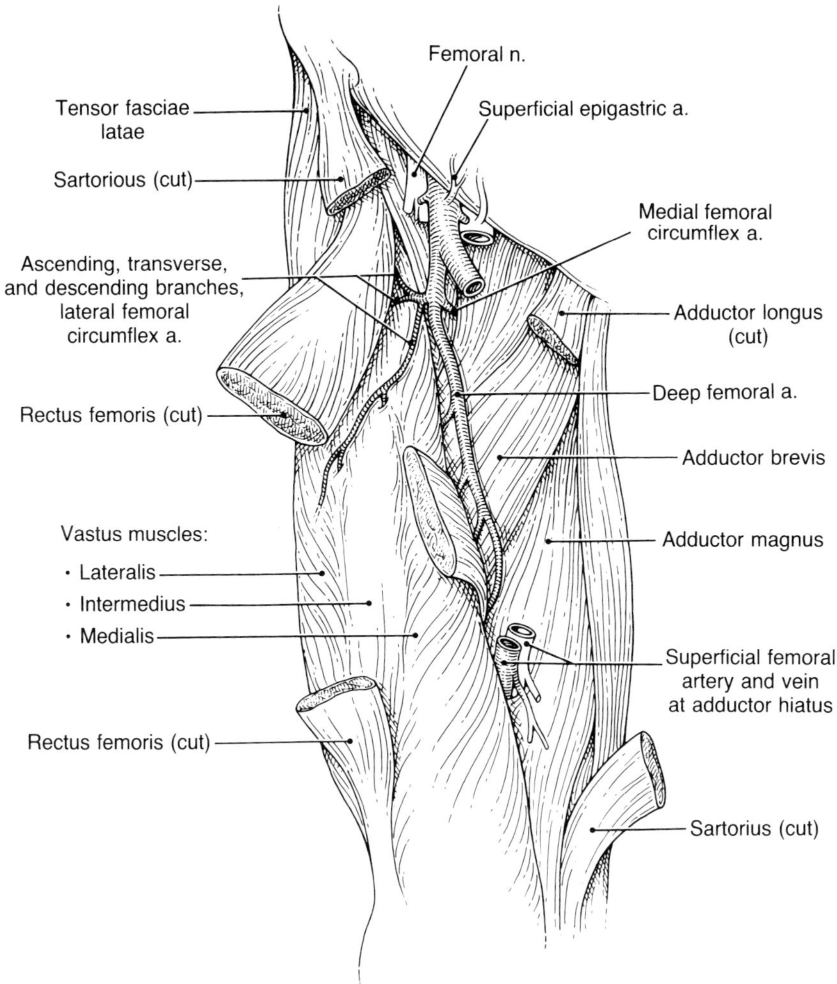

Fig. 4. The adductor longus muscle has been divided, exposing the deep femoral artery (DFA) coursing over the adductor brevis. The first and third perforators arise close to the upper and lower borders of the adductor brevis, while the second arises anterior to the brevis. (Modified from Clemente 1985)

At the apex of the femoral triangle, the deep femoral artery and vein lie directly posterior to the SFA (Basmajian 1971), separated from it by the femoral vein (Henry 1973; Fig. 3). A deep laceration at this level may injure all four vessels, the so-called Butchers block injury.

After crossing the SFA, the DFA continues its descent close to the medial border of the femur, separated from it by the vastus medialis muscle. Passing anterior to the adductor magnus and brevis muscles, it remains deep to the adductor longus (Fig. 4). In the distal one third of the thigh, its terminal branch pierces the adductor magnus close to the femur and is distributed to the hamstring muscles of the posterior thigh (Fig. 5a,b). This terminal portion may be referred to as the fourth perforating branch of the DFA. It anastomoses with the upper branches of the PA (Gray 1985) and tibial recurrent artery (Martin 1972).

Branches of the Deep Femoral Artery

Lateral Femoral Circumflex Artery

The lateral femoral circumflex artery is the largest branch of the DFA. It arises from the lateral aspect, 1.5 cm distal to the origin of the DFA from the CFA (Martin et al. 1968). The lateral circumflex artery arises directly from the CFA in 6%–20% of cases (Gray 1985; Vaas 1975; Woodburne 1983).

From its origin the lateral circumflex artery passes laterally across the iliopsoas and between the branches of the femoral nerve; it then passes dorsal to the sartorius, leaving the femoral triangle deep to the rectus femoris muscles. After giving off branches to the adjacent muscles, it divides into ascending, descending, and transverse branches (Fig. 6).

The ascending branch runs superolaterally, under the tensor fascia lata superficial to the proximal end of the vastus lateralis. It ascends along the trochanteric line of the femur. Inferior to the anterior superior iliac spine it anastomoses with the superficial and deep circumflex iliacs and the iliac branches of the iliofemoral artery (Last 1984). The ascending branch then passes between the gluteus medius and minimus muscles, where it terminates by anastomosing with branches of the superior gluteal artery. It also supplies the adjacent muscles and provides a branch to the front of the hip joint.

The transverse branch is the smallest branch of the lateral circumflex femoral artery and is often absent. It courses laterally over the proximal part of the vastus intermedius, pierces the upper portion of the vastus lateralis, and winds around the femur immediately inferior to the greater trochanter. This branch anastomoses on the back of the thigh the inferior gluteal from above, the medial circumflex medially, and the first perforator from below. This complex forms the "cruciate anastomosis."

The descending branch is a significant distal pathway (Karmody et al. 1987). It slopes inferiorly deep to the rectus femoris in the

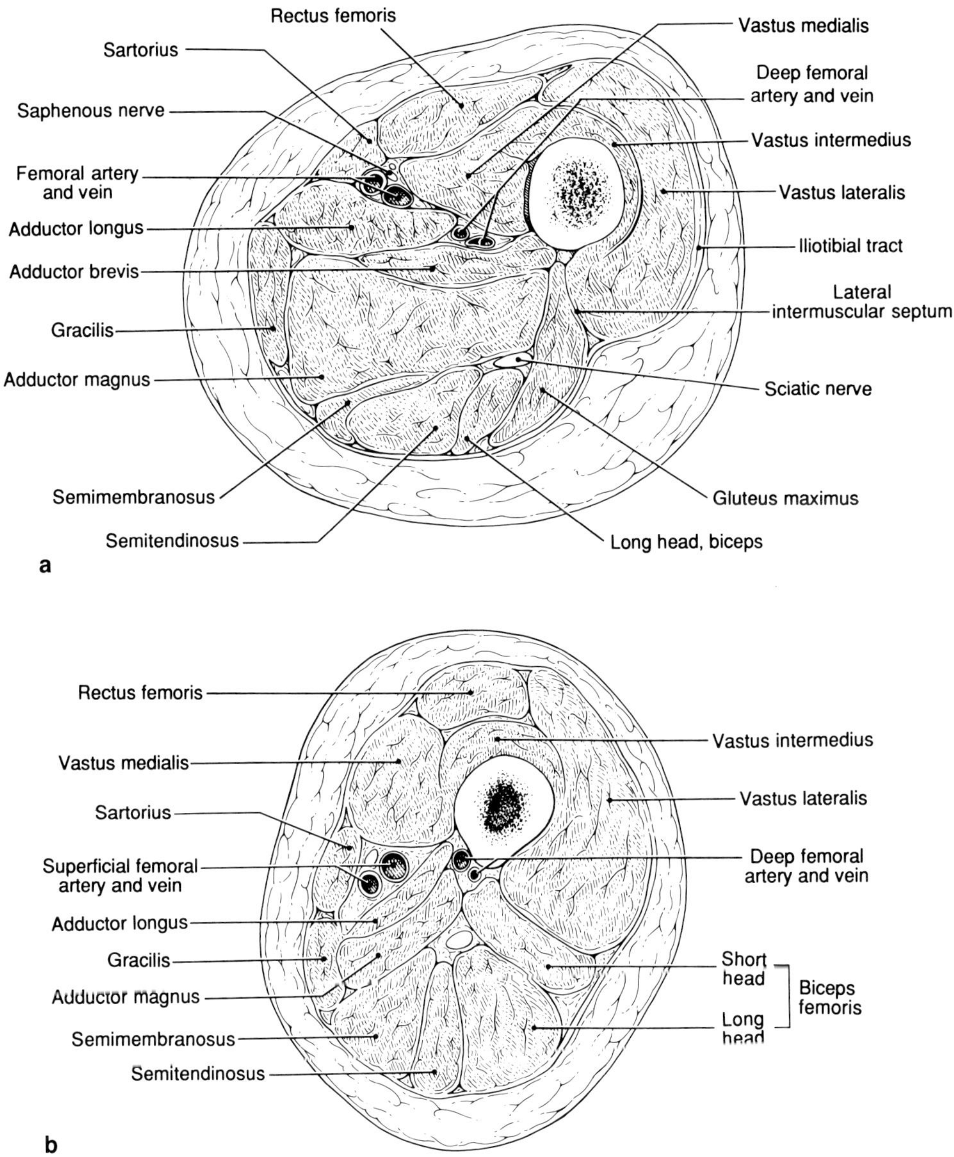

Fig. 5a,b. Transverse sections through the proximal (**a**) and distal (**b**) thigh demonstrate the deep femoral vessels coursing toward the linea aspera of the femur. (Modified from **a** Clemente 1985 and **b** Henry 1973)

groove between vastus lateralis. Numerous branches supply the vastus lateralis as the descending branch passes inferiorly within the muscle, terminating at the knee by an anastomosis with the superior lateral genicular branch of the PA.

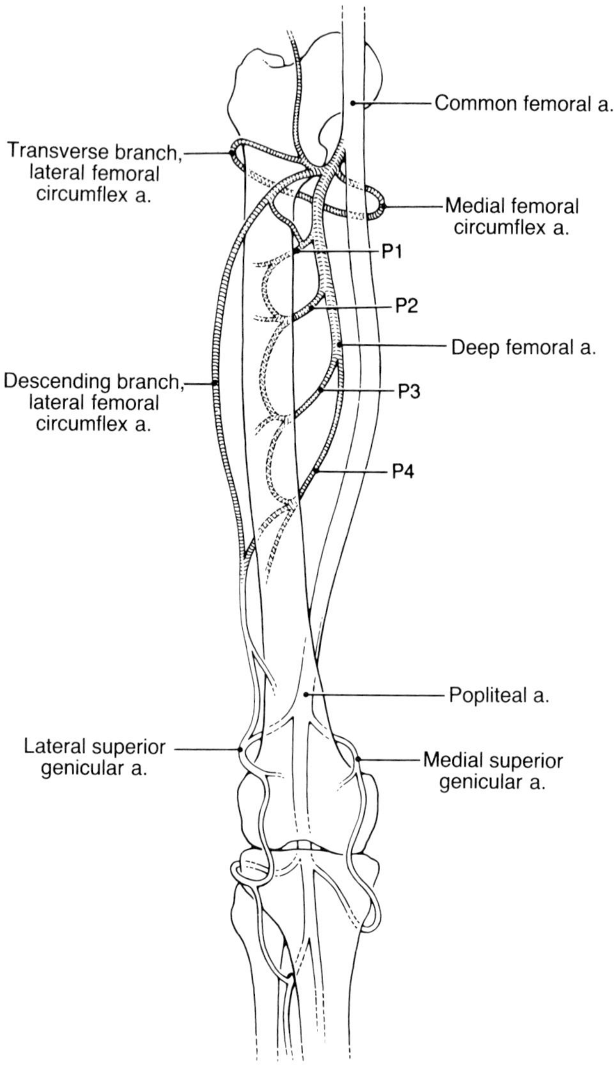

Fig. 6. The lateral femoral circumflex artery is the largest branch of the deep femoral artery (DFA). Through its numerous branches it anastomoses with the pelvic vessels proximally, with the medial femoral circumflex to form the cruciate anastomosis, and via its descending branch with the superior lateral genicular artery at the knee. *P*, pelvic vessel

Variations in the manner of origin of the lateral circumflex artery are fairly common (Figs. 7, 8). Its branches may arise separately from the CFA or DFA (Bergman 1984). The descending branch, in particular, may arise separately, with an independent stem of origin for the ascending and transverse branches.

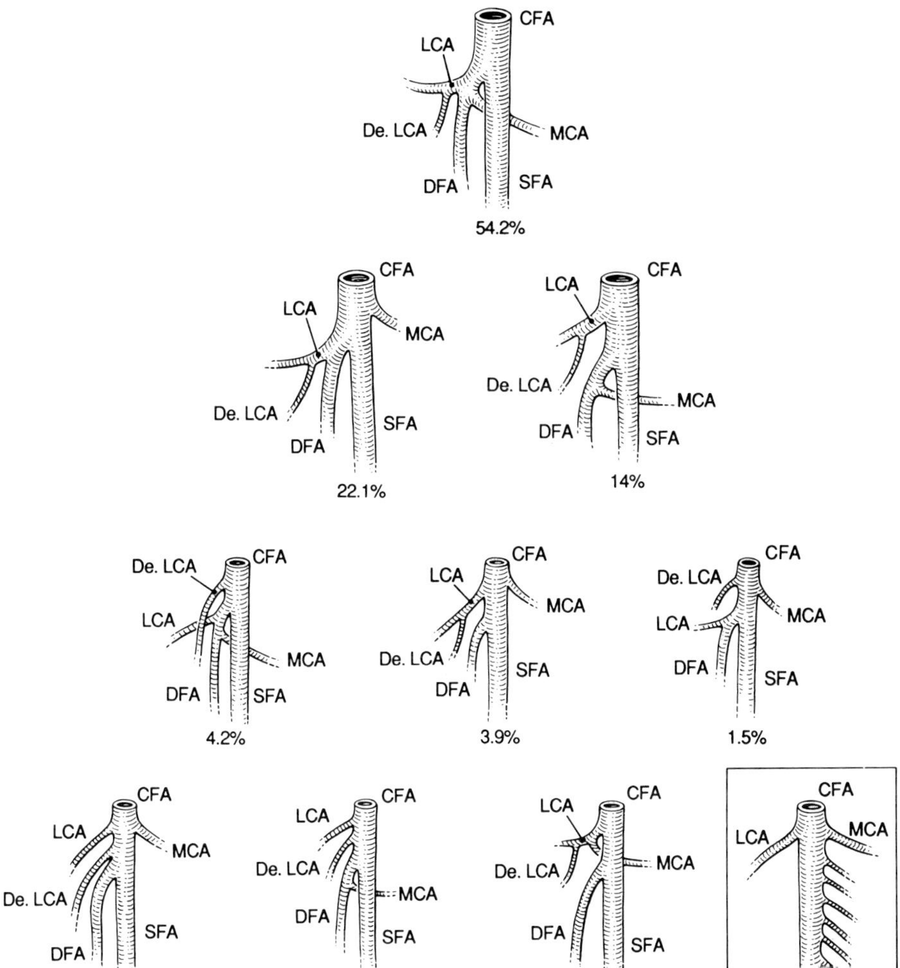

Fig. 7. The varied anatomy of the origin of the circumflex vessels from the deep femoral artery (*DFA*) and the common femoral artery (*CFA*). *SFA*, superficial femoral artery; *LCA*, lateral femoral circumflex artery; *MCA*, medial femoral circumflex artery; *De.*, descending. (Modified from Hollinshead 1969)

Medial Femoral Circumflex Artery (Fig. 9)

The medial femoral circumflex artery originates from the posteromedial aspect of the DFA at or close to the same level as the lateral circumflex artery. In 25%–41% of cases, the medial femoral circumflex artery arises directly from the CFA. It passes posteriorly out of the femoral triangle between the psoas major and pectineus

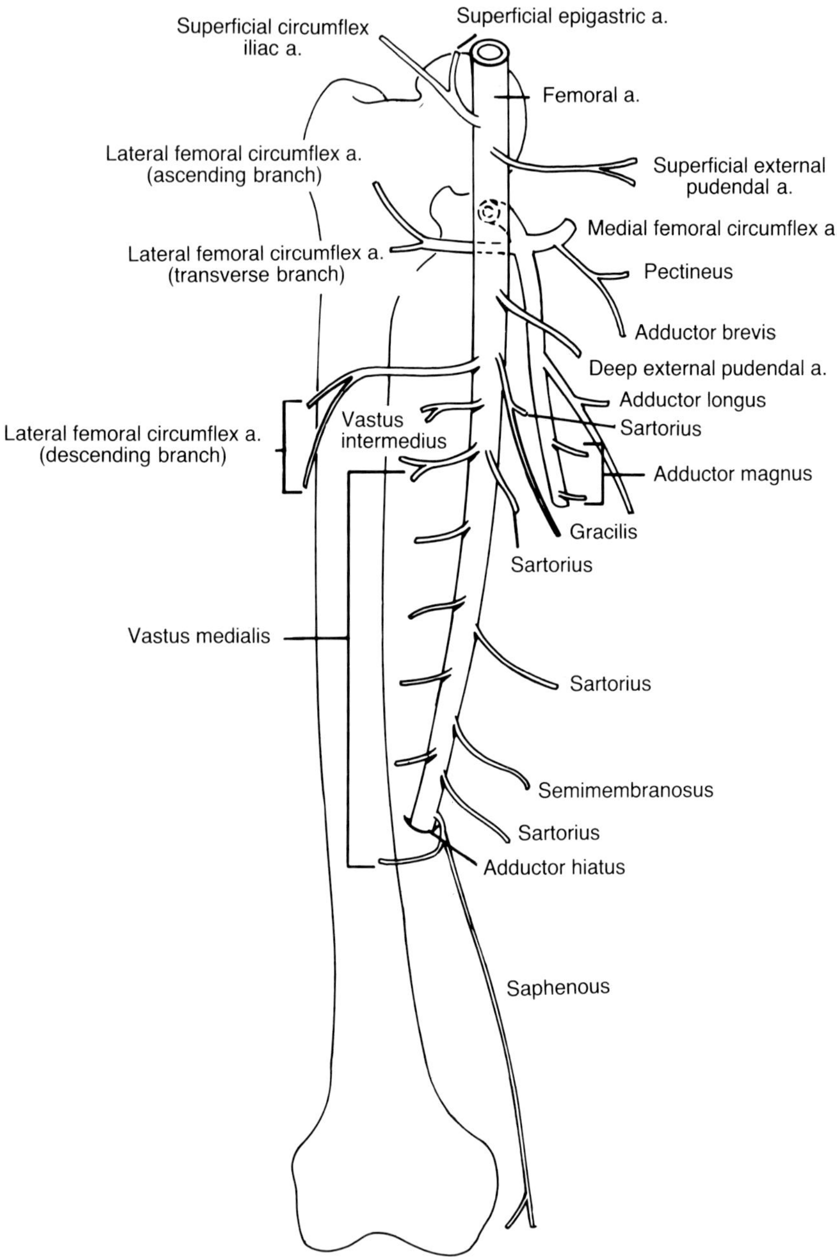

Fig. 8. The rare occurrence of an absent deep femoral artery (DFA). In this situation the circumflex and perforating vessels arise directly from the common femoral channel

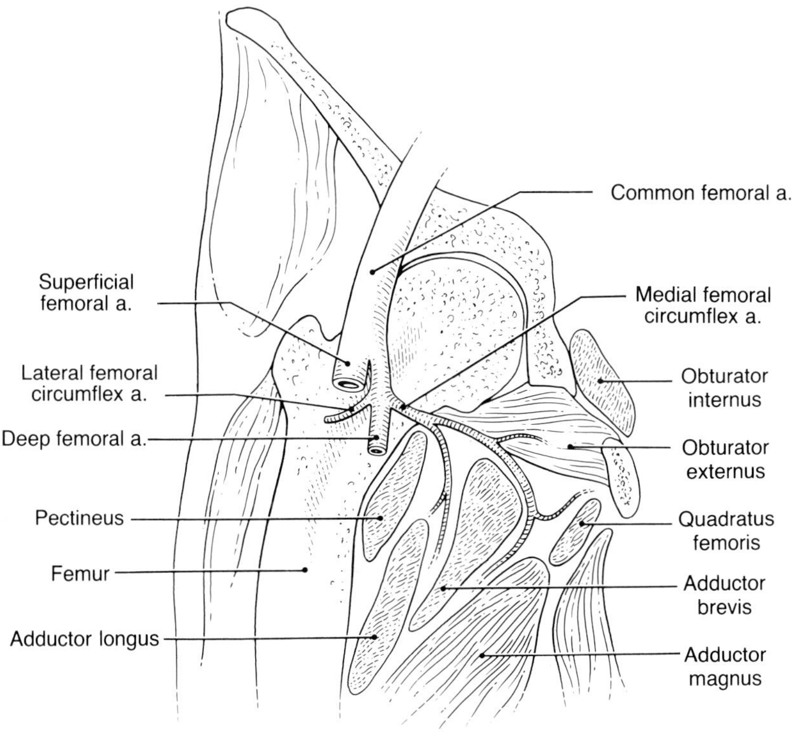

Fig. 9. The medial femoral circumflex artery leaves the femoral triangle by passing deeply between the psoas and pectineus. It then runs between the obturator externus and adductor brevis to reach the interval between the obturator externus and the adductor magnus. There it divides into ascending and transverse branches

muscles under the neck of the femur. Continuing between the obturator externus superiorly and the adductor brevis inferiorly, it reaches the interval between the obturator externus and the adductor magnus, where it divides into ascending and transverse branches. The ascending branch supplies the adductor muscles, the gracilis, and the obturator externus and anastomoses with the obturator artery. The transverse branch descends beneath the adductor brevis, where it supplies both it and the adductor magnus and participates in the cruciate anastomosis.

The medial femoral circumflex artery then continues posteriorly above the iliopsoas insertion, soon dividing into superficial, deep, and acetabular branches. The superficial branch passes between the quadratus femoris and the adductor magnus, thereafter entering the cruciate anastomoses by anastomosing with the inferior gluteal, transverse branch of the DFA.

The deep branch ascends obliquely on the obturator externus, ventral to the quadratus femoris, to the trochanteric fossa, anastomosing with the obturator artery (Romanes 1976), where it communicates with twigs from both gluteal arteries.

The acetabular branch of the medial femoral circumflex artery arises opposite the acetabular notch and enters the hip joint beneath the transverse acetabular ligament. When well developed, it supplies adipose tissue in the acetabular fossa and then courses along the round ligament to the head of the femur. An acetabular branch arises from the medial femoral circumflex artery in 21.3% of cases (Weathersby 1959), and in almost one third of these cases a second acetabular branch arises from an anastomotic connection between the medial circumflex and the obturator artery.

Perforating Branches of the Deep Femoral Artery (Fig. 10)

There are usually three perforating branches which arise from the DFA, although the terminal branch of the DFA is often referred to as the fourth perforating artery. Variably the perforating arteries number from two to six separate branches (Weathersby 1959). These branches provide primary arterial supply to the muscles of the thigh and a large nutrient branch to the femoral shaft.

The term "perforator" was coined because these branches perforate the long tendinous insertion of the adductor magnus to the linea aspera on the back of the femur. Each perforator is protected by a tendinous arch as it passes through the femoral attachments of the adductor magnus. In most cases the perforators arch posteriorly around the femur, ending by piercing the lateral intermuscular septum and assisting supply of the vastus lateralis muscles. Here, at the lateral intermuscular septum, these vessels must be ligated in the posterolateral approach to the femur (Hoppenfield and DeBoer 1984).

The first perforating branch arises above the adductor brevis, the second originates anterior to the adductor brevis, and the third arises inferior to the brevis. Each runs downwards and postero-

Fig. 10. Posterior view of the right thigh before (*above*) and after (*below*) pulling aside the gluteus maximus, long head of biceps, and adductors brevis and magnus to reveal the deep femoral artery (DFA) coursing over the adductor longus and along the linea aspera of the femur. The origins of the perforating vessels are clearly seen

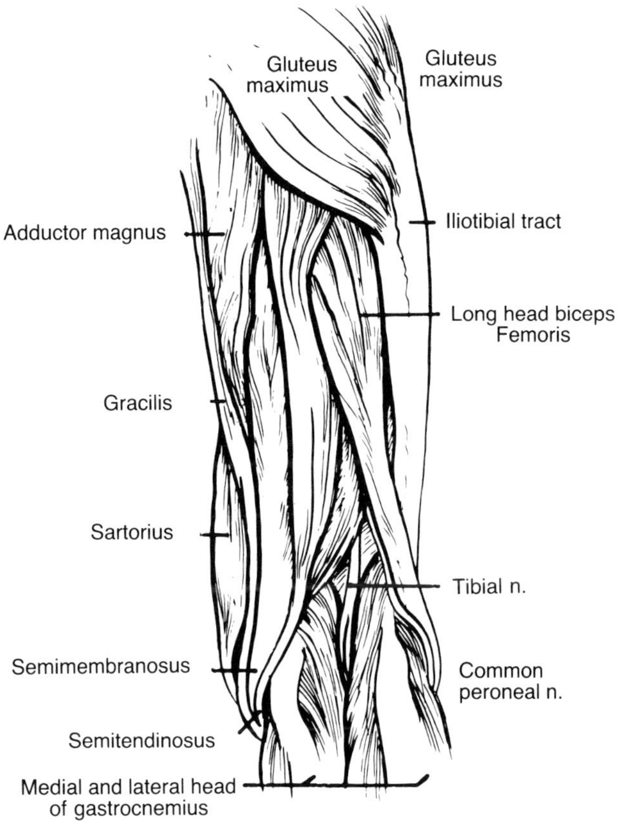
Gluteus maximus
Gluteus maximus
Iliotibial tract
Adductor magnus
Long head biceps Femoris
Gracilis
Sartorius
Tibial n.
Semimembranosus
Common peroneal n.
Semitendinosus
Medial and lateral head of gastrocnemius

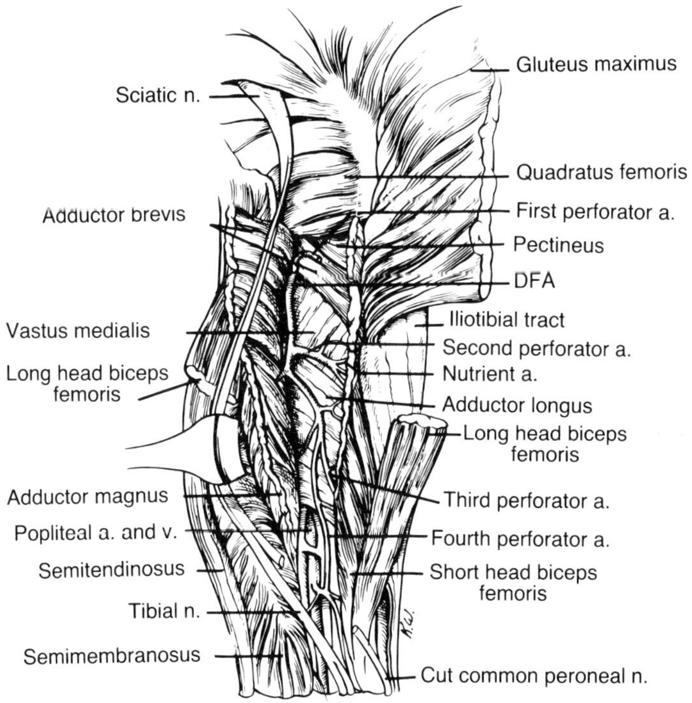
Gluteus maximus
Sciatic n.
Quadratus femoris
First perforator a.
Adductor brevis
Pectineus
DFA
Iliotibial tract
Vastus medialis
Second perforator a.
Long head biceps femoris
Nutrient a.
Adductor longus
Long head biceps femoris
Adductor magnus
Third perforator a.
Popliteal a. and v.
Fourth perforator a.
Semitendinosus
Short head biceps femoris
Tibial n.
Semimembranosus
Cut common peroneal n.

laterally, a feature which helps to distinguish it from the perforating vessels from other medially directed muscular branches.

The first perforating branch passes posteriorly between the pectineus and adductor brevis, occasionally piercing the brevis. A muscular branch leaves the first perforator before it passes deep to the pectineus. This branch commonly passes with the anterior division at the obturator nerve, ramifying then upon the ventral surface of the adductor brevis, supplying the adductor longus before entering the proximal portion of the gracilis.

The first perforating vessel pierces the adductor magnum close to the femur. In its course it supplies the adductor brevis, magnus, long head of the biceps femoris, the semimembranosus, semitendinosus, and the gluteus maximus muscles. It communicates with the inferior gluteal artery, medial and lateral circumflex arteries, and the second perforating artery, the major participants in the cruciate anastomosis. This artery is usually large where it pierces the proximal portion of the adductor magnus near the insertion of the gluteus maximus at the gluteal tuberosity of the femur.

The second perforator is often larger than the first, but occasionally may arise from the DFA along with the first perforator. It runs posteriorly, piercing the tendons of the adductor brevis and magnus. The artery then supplies the long hamstring muscles by ascending and descending branches and then, after providing supply to the short head of the biceps femoris, it pierces the lateral intermuscular septum and enters the vastus lateralis. The ascending and descending branches of the second perforator anastomose freely with the first and third perforators. Typically the nutrient artery to the femur is supplied by the second perforator as it crosses the linea aspera one third to one half of the way along the femoral shaft. The nutrient artery often inclines vertically upwards to enter its bony canal. If, however, there are two nutrient arteries, they usually arise from the first and third perforators.

Occasionally the first two perforating arteries arise from the medial femoral circumflex artery. In these circumstances the DFA forms a single trunk which arises below the lateral femoral circumflex and supplies the lower two perforating arteries (Blankfein 1921).

The third perforating artery arises from the DFA beneath the tendon of adductor longus; it passes posteriorly through the adductor magnus, the short head of the biceps femoris, and then ends in the vastus lateralis. After piercing the adductor magnus, this artery provides branches to the posterolateral muscles and communicates with the second perforating artery proximally and the terminal branch (fourth perforator) distally. Inferiorly it also

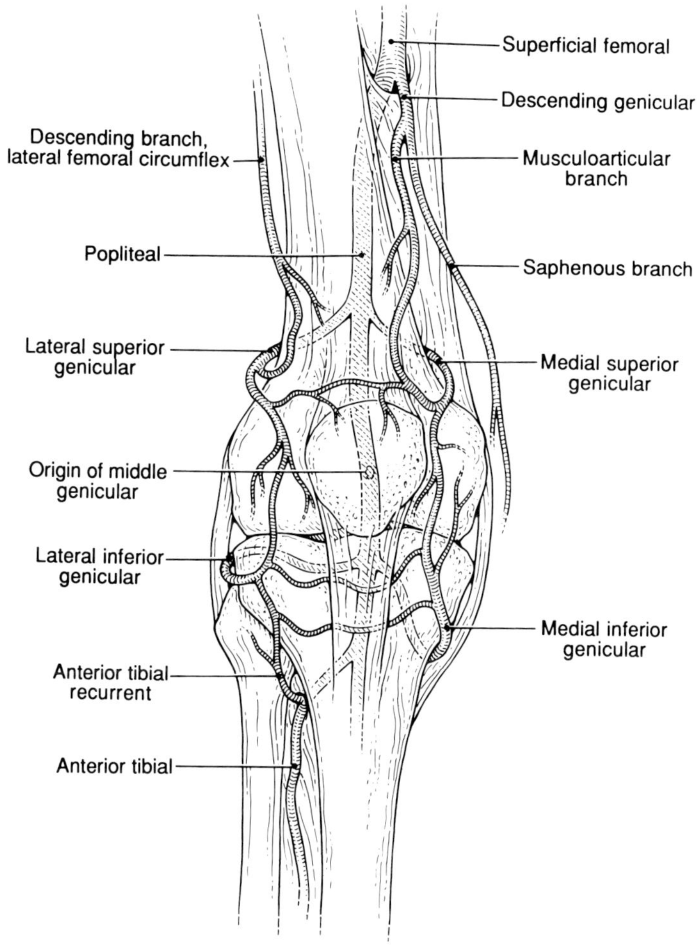

Fig. 11. The rich arterial anastomosis around the knee to which the deep femoral artery (DFA) contributes the descending branch of the lateral circumflex femoral

commonly anastomoses with muscular branches of the PA and may anastomose with branches of the SFA which pass deeply through the adductor magnus proximal to the adductor hiatus.

The fourth perforating artery is usually a small terminal segment of the DFA. This vessel pierces the adductor magnus muscle variably proximal to the level of the hiatus of the adductor magnus. It gives off branches which anastomose with the third perforating artery, muscular branches of the PA, and muscular branches of the SFA. It regularly supplies small twigs to the lower portions of the hamstring muscles and a branch which pierces the short head of the biceps femoris and the vastus lateralis. The SFA may provide a supplemental perforator.

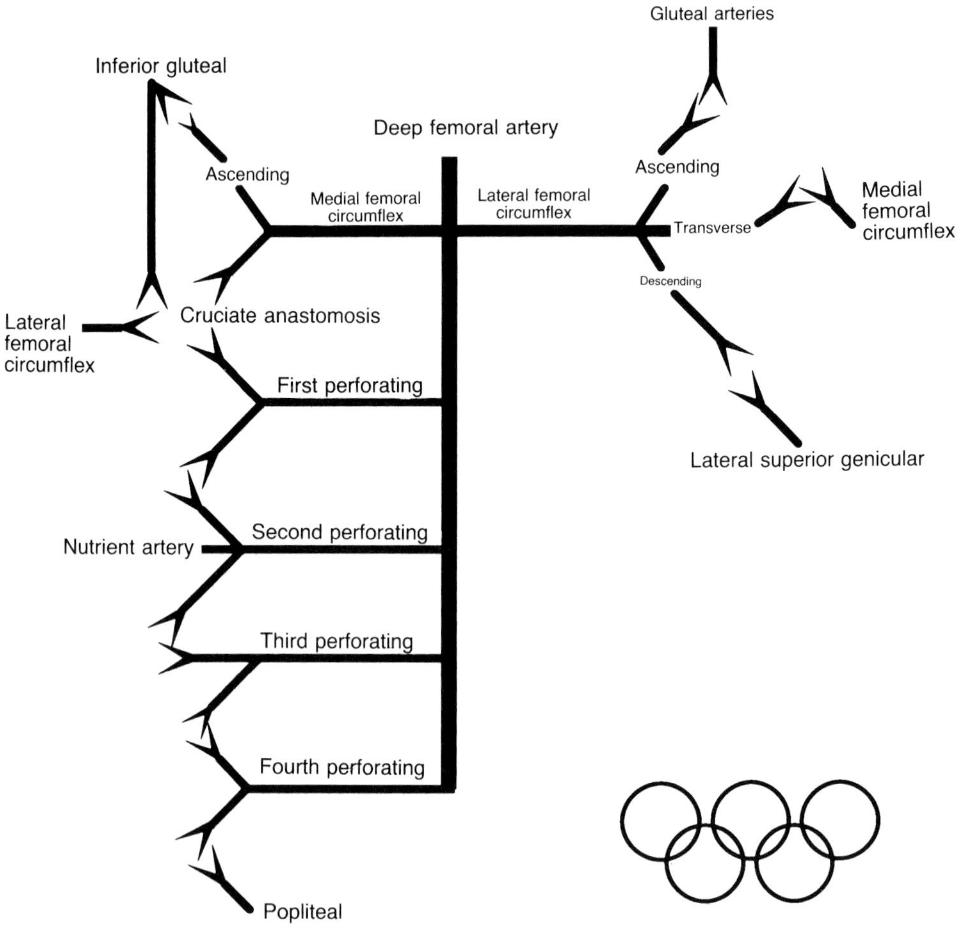

Fig. 12. The longitudinal anastomotic chain between the gluteal arteries of the pelvis via the medial and lateral circumflex arteries to the perforating vessels and finally via the descending branch of the lateral circumflex artery to the superior lateral genicular artery at the knee. The chain of anastomotic *rings* (mnemonically) make the healthy profunda a gold olympic winner

There is, therefore, a longitudinal series of anastomoses down the thigh in the posterior compartment which connect the iliofemoral segment proximally to the PA distally (Feldhaus et al. 1986; Figs. 11, 12). This pathway begins superiorly in the cruciate anastomosis by the interconnections of the inferior gluteal artery with the circumflex arteries and the ascending branch of the first perforator. The sequential perforating branches freely anastomose with one another superficially and adjacent to the linea aspera:

these also anastomose distally with muscular and genicular branches of the PA.

The collective anastomoses form an important collateral pathway in the event of obstruction of the SFA. SFA occlusion is one of the most common findings in patients with vascular disease. Absence of symptoms in many of these patients is testimony to the functional importance of these collateral pathways.

In essence there are three parallel arterial pathways down the leg. These are the SFA, the DFA, and the collateral pathway via the perforators (Waibel and Wolff 1966).

Arterial Blood Supply of the Muscles of the Thigh

Despite the fact that the intramuscular vascular network is diffuse, there may be relatively few anastomoses between the arteries which supply the proximal and distal parts of a given muscle, although the vessels which supply some muscles such as the gluteus maximus have excellent interconnections. Plastic surgeons know this fact better than anyone else and, as a rule, choose selectively only the proximal or distal parts of the muscle as a flap for filling tissue defects, depending upon the more significant source of arterial inflow to the muscle (McCraw 1977; Smet 1989).

Biceps Femoris. The upper two thirds of the muscle are supplied segmentally by perforating branches of the DFA and the lower one third by branches of the PA and distal perforating arteries. These branches are end arteries without significant intramuscular communication: therefore, each deep muscular branch has a specific destiny for a specific part or segment of the muscle. All enter the muscle anteriorly.

Rectus Femoris. The blood supply to the rectus arises proximally by two branches from the lateral circumflex artery. They enter the posterior surface of the muscle 8–10 cm below the inguinal ligament. For all practical purposes the proximal branch supplies the proximal one third of the muscle and the distal branch supplies the distal two thirds.

Gracilis. The proximal two thirds of the gracilis are supplied by branches of the DFA. However, the dominant pedicle arises from the medial circumflex artery. This pedicle is under cover of the adductor longus and pierces the gracilis at the junction of the upper and middle thirds of the thigh, approximately 9–15 cm below the inguinal ligament.

Vastus Lateralis. The descending branch of the lateral femoral circumflex artery supplies the proximal two thirds of the vastus lateralis muscle. Branches originating from the SFA supply the distal one third. Pedicles enter the anterior proximal belly of the muscle located approximately 10 cm below the anterior superior iliac spine.

Tensor Fascia Lata. This muscle is supplied by the ascending branch of the lateral femoral circumflex artery, which enters the muscle 8–10 cm below the anterior superior iliac spine.

Sartorius. This muscle is supplied segmentally by five to six branches originating from the SFA. The intramuscular connections are, however, variable. Consequently, no more than two of the pedicles should be divided when used as a flap. A few small branches originating from the DFA enter the muscle superiorly through its deep surface.

Semimembranosus. The proximal part of this muscle receives blood from branches of the DFA artery which enter the deep surface of the muscle 10 cm inferior to the ischial tuberosity. Branches from the SFA supply the distal portion of the muscle.

Gluteus Maximus. This larger muscle is supplied predominantly by the superior and inferior gluteal arteries. Excellent intramuscular communications exist.

Vastus Medialis. Segmental branches arising from the DFA supply the proximal one third of the vastus medialis. The remainder is supplied by the SFA.

Veins

The deep femoral vein most frequently lies posteromedial to the artery and drains to the common femoral. It usually receives two or three branches: the superficial external iliac vein and one or two quadriceps veins. The medial and lateral circumflex veins, however, generally drain directly to the common femoral. The deep femoral enters the common femoral vein at a more variable level than the corresponding arteries. The most common arrangement is for the deep femoral vein to drain into the common femoral approximately 8 cm (range, 5–15 cm) below the inguinal ligament (Edwards and Robuck 1947).

The lateral circumflex vein is an important landmark. It crosses the angle between the DFA and SFA to reach the common femoral vein. It therefore marks the DFA and is easily injured during its dissection.

Each perforating artery is accompanied by two "venae comitantes"; these drain to the deep femoral vein.

A relatively common variation in the venous anatomy is a large communication between the inferior end of the profunda vein and either the popliteal vein or the superficial femoral vein (Mavor and Galloway 1967). Another variant is for the popliteal vein to divide into two trunks, one of which flows into the deep femoral while the other drains into the superficial femoral vein.

Occasionally there may not be a vein which corresponds to the DFA, in which case numerous branches occur which cross the DFA anteriorly, draining into the superficial or common femoral vein directly.

References

Anderson J (ed) Grant's atlas of anatomy, 9th edn. Williams and Wilkins, Baltimore

Basmajian JV (1971) Method of anatomy; by regions, descriptive and deductive. Williams and Wilkins, Baltimore, pp 309–319

Beales JS, Adcock FA, Frawley JS, Nathan BE, Maclachan MSF, Martin P, Steiner RE (1971) The radiological assessment of disease of the profunda femoris artery. Br J Radiol 44: 854–859

Bergman RA, Thompson SA, Afifi AK (1984) Catalog of human variation. Urban and Schwarzenberg, Baltimore, pp 125–128

Blankfein E (1921) An example of dissociation of the branches of the A. profunda femoris. Anat Rec Phila XXI: 329

Chleborad WP, Dawson DL (1990) The profunda femoris artery: variations and clinical applications. Clin Anat 3: 33–40

Clemente CD (ed) (1985) Gray's anatomy of the human body, 30th edn. Lea and Febiger, Philadelphia

Cunningham DJ (1981) Cunningham's textbook of anatomy, 12th edn. Oxford University Press, Oxford, pp 936–938

Edwards EA, Robuck JD (1947) Applied anatomy of femoral vein and its tributaries. Surg Gynecol Obstet 85: 547–557

Feldhaus RJ, Sterpetti AV, Schultz RD, Peetz DJ (1986) A technique for profunda femoris artery reconstruction: hemodynamic assessment and functional results. Ann Surg 203: 390–398

Haimovici (1984) Vascular surgery: principles and techniques, 2nd edn. Appleton-Century-Crofts, Norwalk, pp 537–546

Henry AK (1973) Extensile exposure, 2nd edn. Churchill Livingstone, Edinburgh, pp 227–241

Hershey FB, Auer AI (1974) Extended surgical approach to the profunda femoris artery. Surg Gynecol Obstet 138: 88–90

Hollinshead WH (1969) Anatomy for surgeons, vol 3, 2nd edn. Harper and Row, New York, pp 575–589

Hoppenfeld S, DeBoer P (1984) Surgical exposures in orthopaedics: the anatomic approach. Lippincott, Philadelphia, pp 380–400

Johnston TB (1912) A rare anomaly of the a. profunda femoris. Anat Anz 42: 269–272

Karmody AM, Leather RP, Corson JD, Shah DM (1987) Surgery of the profunda femoris artery. In: Wilson SE, Veith FJ, Hobson RW, Williams RA (eds) Vascular surgery principles and practice. McGraw Hill, New York, pp 425–436

Last RJ (1984) Anatomy: regional and applied, 7th edn. Churchill Livingstone, Edinburgh, pp 130–145

Leeds FH, Gilfillan RS (1961) Importance of profunda femoris artery in the revascularization of the ischemic limb. Arch Surg 82: 25–31

Martin P (1972) A reconsideration of arterial reconstruction below the inguinal ligament. J Cardiovasc Surg 13: 24–29

Martin P, Jamieson C (1974) The rationale for and measurement after profundoplasty. Surg Clin North Am 54: 95–109

Martin P, Renwick S, Stephenson C (1968) On the surgery of the profunda femoris artery. Br J Surg 55: 539–542

Martin P, Frawley JE, Barabas AP, Rosengarten DS (1972) On the surgery of atherosclerosis of the profunda femoris artery. Surgery 71: 182–189

Mavor GE, Galloway JM (1967) Collaterals of the deep venous circulation of the lower limb. Surg Gynecol Obstet 125: 561–571

McCraw JB (1977) Reconstructive plastic surgery. Saunders, Philadelphia, pp 3560–3563

Morris GC Jr, Edwards E, Cooley DA, Crawford ES, De Bakey ME (1961) Surgical importance of profunda femoris artery: analysis of 102 cases with combined aortoiliac and femoropopliteal occlusive disease treated by revascularization of deep femoral artery. Arch Surg 82: 32–37

Romanes GJ (1976) Upper and lower limbs. In: Cunnigham DJ, Romanes GJ (eds) Cunningham's manual of practical anatomy, vol 1, 14th edn. University Press, New York, pp 112–115

Schoeffer JP (1942) Morris human anatomy, 11th edn. Blakiston, New York, pp 611–828

Schrutz A (1894) Zu Zaaijers artikel: seltene Abweichung der A. profunda femoris. Anat Anz 9: 727

Siddharth P, Smith NL, Mason RA, Giron F (1985) Variational anatomy of the deep femoral artery. Anat Rec 212: 206–209

Skandalakis JE (1980) The rape of anatomy. Am Surg 46: 197–200

Skandalakis JE (1984) The incompetent professor of anatomy in the United States. Anat Clin 6: 227–228

Skandalakis JE, Gray SW (1969) The very unpopular science. Surg Gynecol Obstet 128: 350–357

Skandalakis JE, Gray SW (1983) Anatomy: a prometheus bound 146: 291–292
Skandalakis JE, Rowe JS Jr, Gray SW (1974) Editorial: surgical anatomy. Surgery 75: 148–149
Smet HT (1989) Tissue transfers in reconstructive surgery. Raven, New York, pp 155–174
Vaas F (1975) Some considerations concerning the deep femoral artery. Arch Chir Neerl 27: 25–34
Waibel P, Wolff G (1966) The collateral circulation in occlusions of the femoral artery: an experimental study. Surgery 60: 912–918
Weathersby HT (1959) The origin of the artery of the ligamentum teres femoris. J Bone Joint Surg [Am] 41A: 261–263
Woodburne RT (1983) Essentials of human anatomy, 7th edn. Oxford University Press, New York, pp 523–557

2 Embryology and Phylogenetic Considerations

F. VAAS and R.J.A.M. VAN DONGEN

Embryology

In the early decades of this century some experimental research was carried out, allowing good insight into the embryonic development of the arterial system of the lower extremity. It was demonstrated that the first vessels develop from a preexisting vascular network (Evans 1909). These join to form several vascular trunks of different caliber (Senior 1919; Greebe 1977, 1989).

From the umbilical artery, which originates from the dorsal aorta, a branch develops, called the axial artery (Fig. 1). This vessel runs down on the dorsal side of the pelvis lateral to the sciatic nerve. It must be regarded as the embryonic main artery of the lower extremity. At a later stage, three parts of this axial artery can be distinguished: a proximal part, the sciatic artery, a middle part at the level of the knee, called the deep popliteal artery, and a distal segment, the embryonic interosseous artery. Later, the external iliac artery (EIA) sprouts from the umbilical artery proximal to the origin of the axial artery.

From the EIA the inferior epigastric artery and the proximal part of the femoral artery develop (Fig. 2). The middle part of the femoral artery comes into existence by the development of a big trunk, which evolves from the ventrally located femoral network, called the rete femorale. Its distal portion develops from the superior communicating ramus, a branch of the sciatic artery, running back from the level of the hiatus tendineus.

From the rete femorale arises a second large branch, the deep femoral artery (DFA; Fig. 3). Its terminal branches form the network of the sciatic artery. Simultaneously with the development of the femoral vessels, the greater part of the sciatic artery disappears (Fig. 3). The proximal part continues to exist as the inferior gluteal artery. Also one of the branches of the inferior gluteal artery, the concomitant ramus of the sciatic artery may be considered as a remnant of the sciatic artery. Later on, the

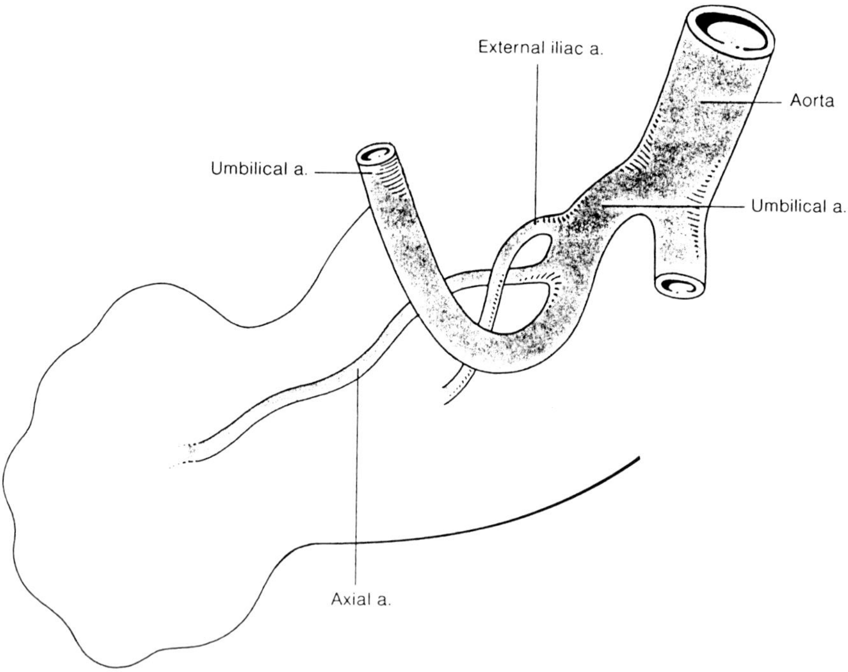

Fig. 1. Evolution of the axial and external iliac arteries from the umbilical artery

embryonic deep popliteal artery develops into the proximal portion of the adult popliteal artery.

Following birth, as soon as blood circulation through the placenta is interrupted, the caliber of the internal iliac artery (IIA) decreases. Thereafter, the EIA is the direct continuation of the common iliac artery (CIA).

Phylogenetic Considerations

In operations on the DFA, the large caliber of this artery is a striking finding. This situation, frequently so beneficial to the patient with an occlusion of the superficial femoral artery (SFA), can be explained by studying the literature concerning the pattern of vascularization of the posterior extremities of higher vertebrate animals (Herrmann 1940; Bickhardt 1961; Ghoshal and Getty 1967; Ghoshal 1972; Vaas 1975).

In all these vertebrates, the DFA originates from the iliac artery proximal to the site where this vessel leaves the pelvis

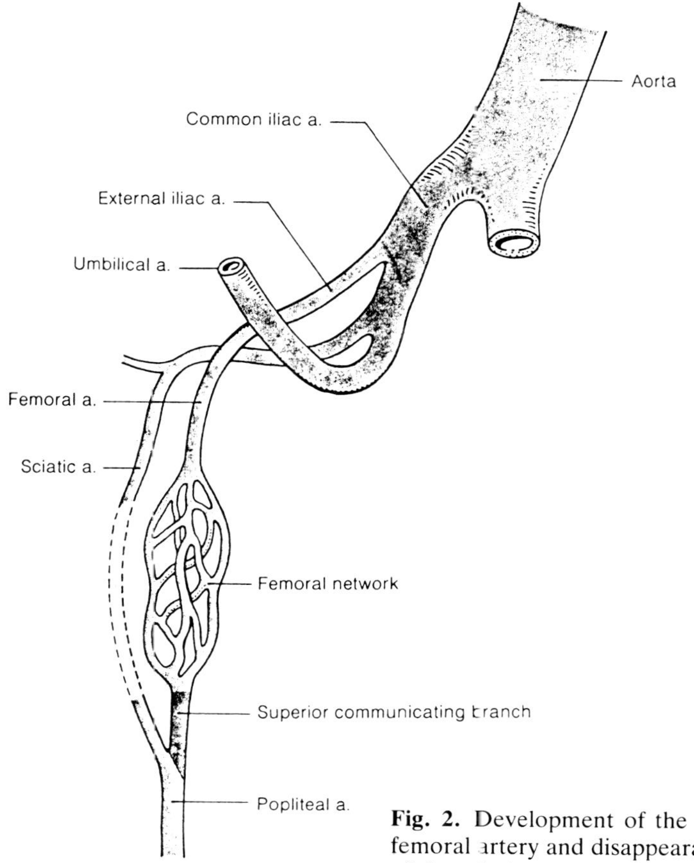

Fig. 2. Development of the ilio-femoral artery and disappearance of the sciatic artery

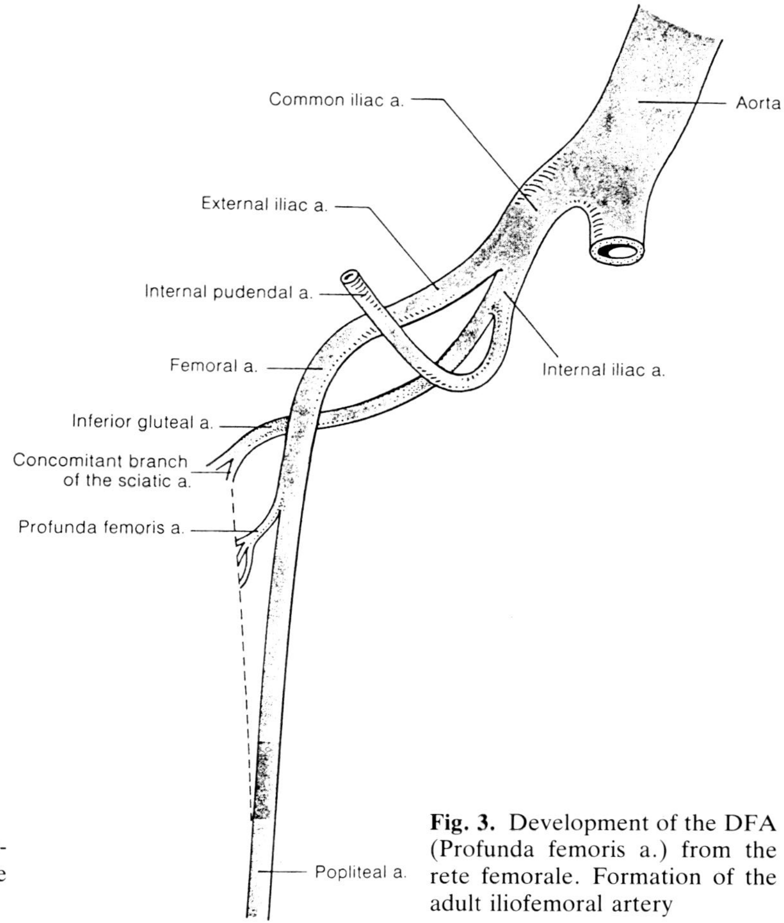

Fig. 3. Development of the DFA (Profunda femoris a.) from the rete femorale. Formation of the adult iliofemoral artery

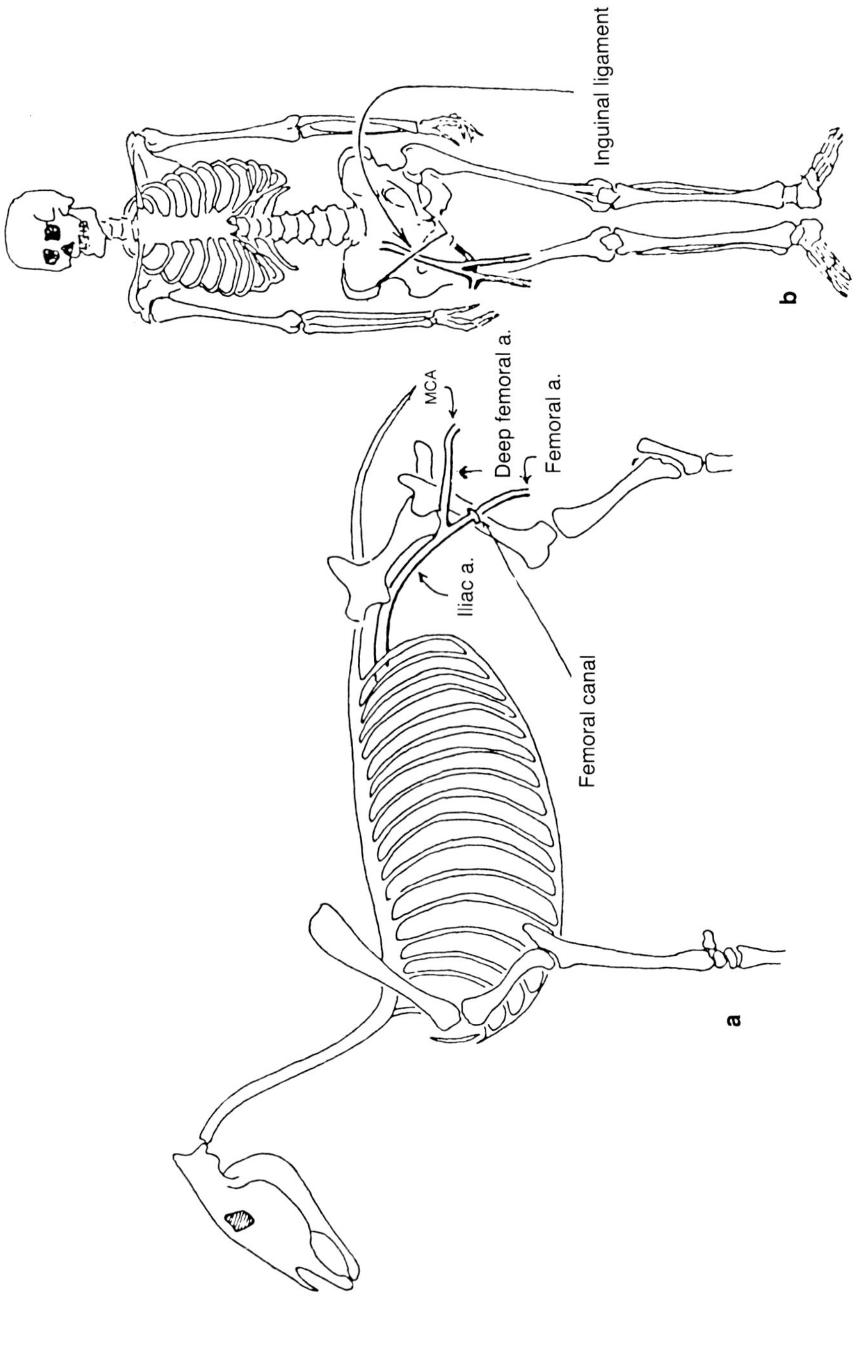

Fig. 4. **a** Vascularization of the posterior extremity in vertebrate animals. The deep femoral artery (DFA) is a pelvic artery. *MCA*, medial femoral circumflex artery. **b** Vascularization of the lower extremity in man. The DFA is a limb artery

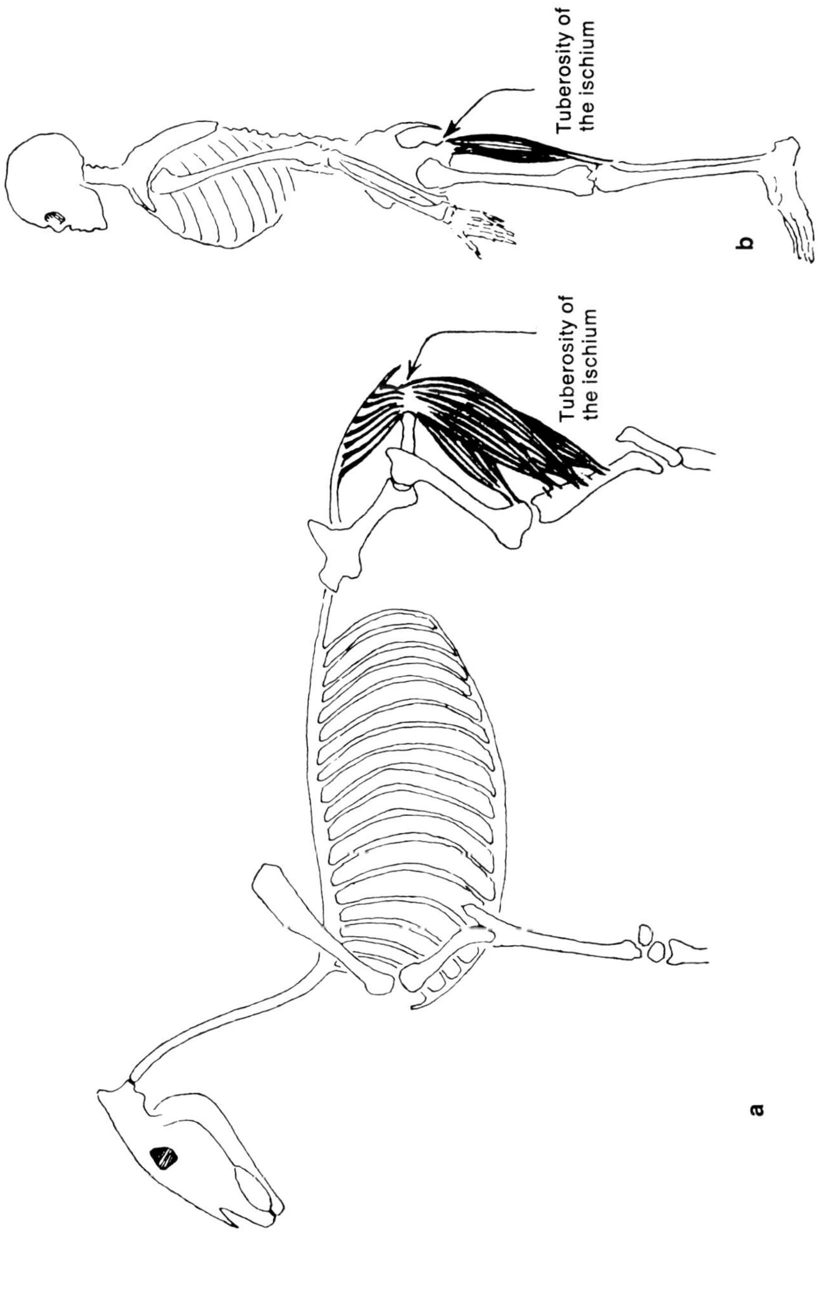

Fig. 5. a Extensors of the posterior extremity in vertebrate animals. **b** Extensors of the lower extremity in man

through the femoral canal, where it becomes the femoral artery. Accordingly, in the vertebrates, the DFA is a pelvic artery (Fig. 4). A constant branch of this artery is the medial femoral circumflex artery. In animals, the DFA and the medial femoral circumflex artery supply blood to, amongst others, the semimembranosus, the semitendinosus, and the biceps femoris muscles. In humans, these muscles are attached to the tuberosity of the ischium. In other vertebrates, however, they insert not only onto the tuberosity of the ischium, but also onto the caudal portion of the spinal column (Fig. 5). Moreover, these extensor muscles are much more developed, enabling the animal to run fast and to jump far. Accordingly, the DFA and the medial circumflex femoral artery have a large caliber in these animals.

In humans, with their upright posture, the extensor and adductor muscles of the thigh are much less well developed. Furthermore, we observe that the DFA is not a branch of the iliac artery, but originates distal to the inguinal ligament from the common femoral artery (CFA). It is a limb artery (Fig. 4). Nevertheless, in humans the DFA has a large caliber. Its phylogenesis provides an explanation for this fact.

References

Bickhardt K (1961) Arterien und Venen der Hintergliedmasse des Schweines. Thesis, Hannover

Evans HM (1909) On the development of the aorta, cardinal and umbilical veins and the other blood vessels of vertebral embryos from capillaries. Anat Rec 3: 498–511

Ghoshal NG (1972) The arteries of the pelvic limb of the cat (Felis domesticus). Zentralbl Veterinaermed 19: 78–85

Ghoshal NG, Getty R (1967) The arterial supply of the appendages of the goat. Veterinarian 29: 123–127

Greebe J (1977) Congenital anomalies of the iliofemoral artery. J Cardiovasc Surg 18: 317–323

Greebe J (1989) Congenital malformations of the iliofemoral artery. In: Heberer G, van Dongen RJAM, Aigner K (eds) Vascular surgery. Springer, Berlin Heidelberg New York, pp 216–222

Herrmann G (1940) Ueber die Arterien der Hintergliedmasse des Hundes. Thesis, Hannover

Senior HD (1919) The development of the arteries of the human lower extremity. Am J Anat 25: 55–61

Vaas F (1975) Some considerations concerning the deep femoral artery. Arch Chir Neerl 27: 25–34

3 Atherosclerotic Lesions of the Deep Femoral Artery – Profundapopliteal Collateral System

F. Vaas and R.J.A.M. van Dongen

Distribution of Atherosclerotic Lesions

Surgery of the deep femoral artery (DFA) requires good knowledge of the distribution of atherosclerotic lesions of the common femoral artery's (CFA) bifurcation and the DFA.

Many vascular surgeons assert that the DFA – being a so-called supply artery – is affected very little by atherosclerosis, in contrast to the superficial femoral artery (SFA), which in its role as a transport artery is supposed to be more frequently and more severely affected. Moreover, it is generally assumed that atherosclerotic narrowing of the DFA is limited to the proximal part. On the whole, these concepts are right, but there are many exceptions. Arteriographic studies and observations during surgery reveal in many cases severe atherosclerotic lesions of the trunk and distal portion of the DFA.

The reverse applies to the SFA. An arteriographically established occlusion of the SFA is often supposed to be due to arteriosclerosis. In many cases, however, the walls of the proximal part of this are free from arteriosclerotic lesions. The occlusion of the SFA is caused by the proximal extension of a thrombus due to an occlusion at the level of Hunter's canal, where the attachment of the artery to the tendon of the adductor magnus muscle brings about severe lesions on the inner aspect of this artery. In such circumstances arteriography is misleading and gives the erroneous impression that the entire SFA is obstructed due to arteriosclerosis. In many cases, the DFA is more severely affected by atherosclerosis than is the SFA.

This controversy prompted us some years ago to make a study of the distribution of atherosclerotic lesions of the arteries near the femoral bifurcation (Vaas 1982).

In 100 unselected corpses of patients over 45 years of age (56 men and 44 women), the femoral bifurcation was removed. Five sections were made of each specimen (Fig. 1):

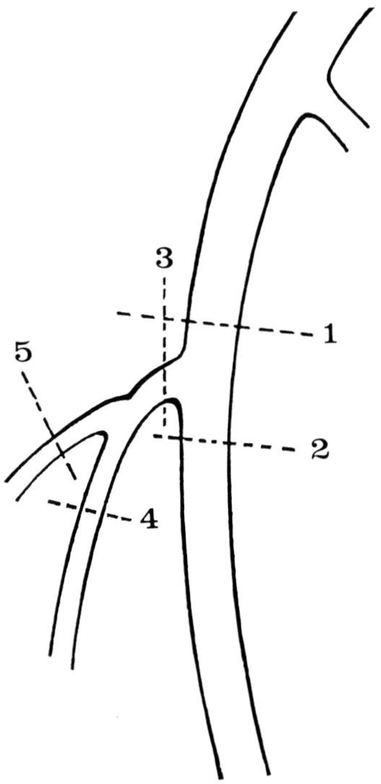

Fig. 1. The five sections of the specimens. See text for details

1. Of the CFA 1 cm proximal to the bifurcation (X_1)
2. Of the SFA 1 cm distal to the bifurcation (X_2)
3. Of the DFA at the level of its takeoff (X_3)
4. Of the DFA 2 cm below the origin of the lateral femoral circumflex artery (X_4)
5. Of the lateral femoral circumflex artery 1 cm beyond its origin (X_5)

All these sections were stained according to the Van Giesen method for impregnating elastin. For each specimen, the five sections were represented schematically on millimeter graph paper and the number of squares within the circle indicating the circumference of the vessel as well as the number of squares within the narrowed area were counted. The cross-sectional area of the open lumen divided by that of the total vessel yield a percentage that expresses the degree of narrowing of each section. The diagrams in Figs. 2 and 3 give examples.

If the generally accepted opinion is correct, the difference in the mean percentages of narrowing of sections 2 and 4 should be positive, as should be the difference between sections 3 and 4.

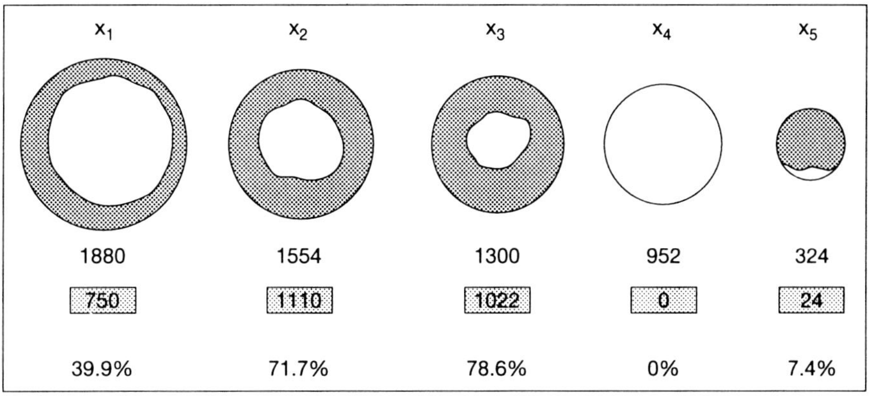

Fig. 2. Considerable narrowing of the proximal deep femoral artery (DFA, X_3) and the superficial femoral artery (SFA, X_2) due to atherosclerosis. More distally (X_4), the DFA is not affected by atherosclerosis

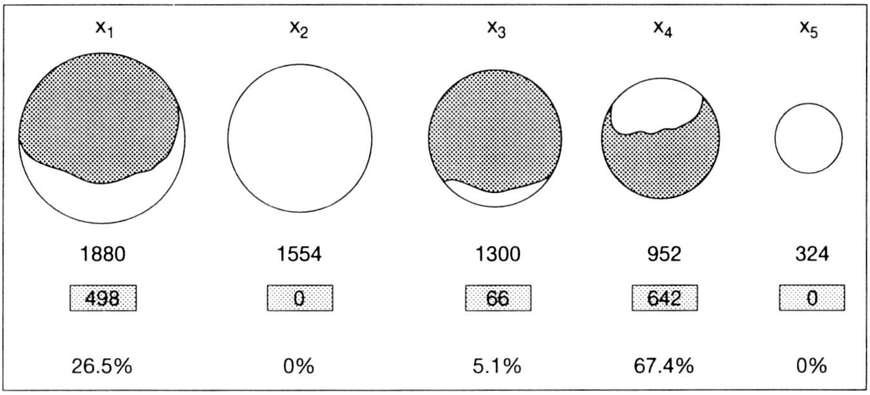

Fig. 3. The superficial femoral artery (SFA, X_2), the transport artery, is free from atherosclerotic lesions. Slight narrowing of the deep femoral artery (DFA) at its origin (X_3). More distally, the DFA (X_4) is severely narrowed by atherosclerosis

Table 1 shows that the percentages of narrowing in all arteries are substantially higher in men than in women. Also, the standard deviation is often large in relation to the mean, which is due to a few specimens with a high degree of narrowing. However, this is not typically related to any particular site.

Table 2 shows an analysis of the differences in percentages of narrowing at the various sites. In only four cases does the mean difference differ significantly from zero. However, in these cases

Table 1. Mean and standard deviation (SD) of the percentages of narrowing for each of the five sections

Section		Men		Women	
		Mean (%)	SD (%)	Mean (%)	SD (%)
Common femoral artery	(X_1)	26	14	16	12
Superficial femoral artery	(X_2)	27	25	16	23
Deep femoral artery (bifurcation)	(X_3)	30	21	12	13
Deep femoral artery	(X_4)	22	20	15	17
Lateral femoral circumflex artery	(X_5)	23	22	10	15

Table 2. Analysis of differences in the percentages of narrowing at the five sites X_1–X_5

Two sites compared	Men		Women	
	Mean (%)	SD (%)	Mean (%)	SD (%)
X_1-X_2	−0.1	20	−0.2	20
X_1-X_3	−3.2	18	3.9*	12
X_1-X_4	4.4	22	0.9	17
X_1-X_5	3.3	23	5.3*	15
X_2-X_3	−3.1	27	4.1	19
X_2-X_4	4.5	32	1.1	20
X_2-X_5	3.4	32	5.5	20
X_3-X_4	7.5*	27	−2.9	18
X_3-X_5	6.5*	22	1.5	17
X_4-X_5	−1.0	27	4.4	20

* Significant at the 5% level (Student's *t* test for paired observations).

also, a considerable proportion showed a negative difference, and another considerable proportion a positive difference. In other words, for no two sites is the narrowing in one site systematically more severe than in the other.

King et al. (1984) carried out an arteriographic study to quantify arteriosclerotic involvement of the DFA. Broadly, they found the same overall results, but in comparing patients with and without diabetes it was noted that patients with diabetes exhibited a significantly higher incidence and severity of lesions in the middle and distal portions of the DFA trunk than patients without diabetes.

With regard to the problem considered, the following three conclusions can be drawn:

1. Atherosclerosis does not cause significantly more narrowing in the proximal segment of the SFA (section 2 in the list above) than in the distal part of the CFA (section 1) or in the segment of the DFA situated 2 cm distal to the origin of the lateral femoral circumflex artery (section 4).
2. In the majority of cases, the obstructing lesions extend a substantial distance down into the trunk of the DFA. In men, the origin of the DFA (section 3) is narrowed more than the part of this artery situated further distally (section 4), to a statistically significant extent. In women, on the other hand, there is no significant difference.
3. Patients without diabetes more frequently have disease limited to the DFA orifice and the circumflex vessels; patients with diabetes are prone to extensive DFA involvement.

These findings indicate that especially in diabetic patients a profundaplasty should not be limited to the first few centimeters of this artery on the assumption that further downstream the atherosclerotic thickening of the wall is not of importance. This vessel should be exposed down and widened over a distance of at least 8–10 cm.

The same applies to revascularization procedures of the DFA. In most cases, the distal anastomosis will have to be created at the level of the first or second perforating branch.

Our study shows that arteriosclerotic lesions are distributed over the femoral bifurcation and the DFA in a highly bizarre pattern. The concept that artherosclerosis mainly affects the transport artery, i.e., the SFA, and spares the supply artery, i.e., the DFA, proves to be untenable.

Profundapopliteal Collateral System

The DFA and the SFA develop from the same embryonic system, the rete femorale. From an embryologic point of view, a coherence between DFA and SFA exists. This coherence is expressed when the SFA is occluded in adults. Under these circumstances two main groups of branches of the DFA, i.e., the femoral circumflex arteries and the perforating branches, both of them developed from the

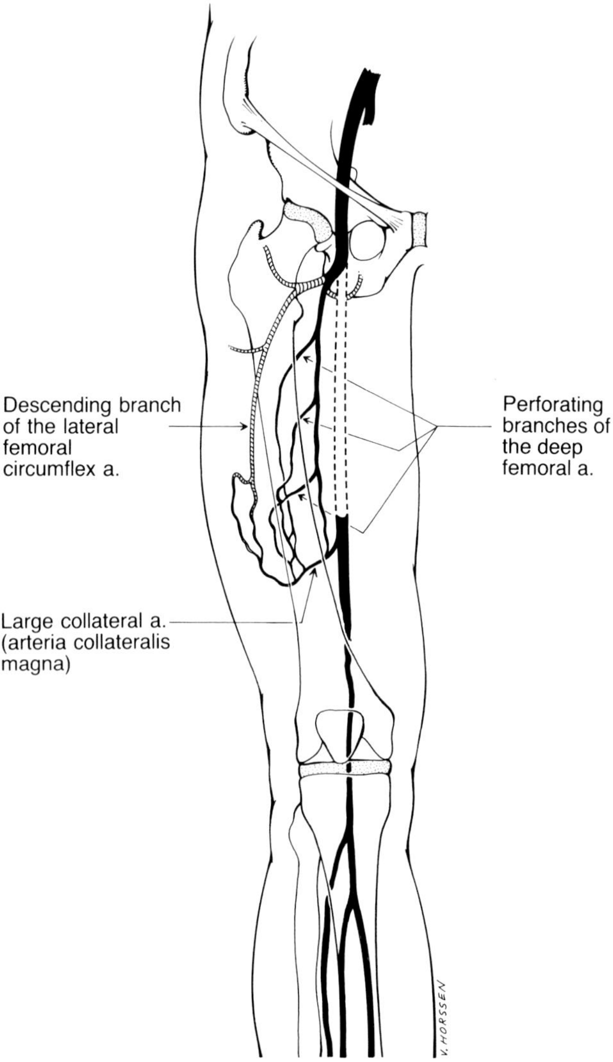

Fig. 4. In occlusion of the superficial femoral artery (SFA), the main groups of branches of the deep femoral artery (DFA), i.e., the femoral circumflex arteries and the perforating branches form a detour for bypassing the obstruction

sciatic and femoral networks and both of them anastomosing with branches of the popliteal artery (PA), function as collaterals: the profundapopliteal collateral system (Fig. 4).

Of the two circumflex arteries, the lateral femoral circumflex artery is the more important and more constant source of the profundapopliteal collaterals. The well-developed descending branch of this artery anastomoses via the lateral superior genicular branch of the PA with the rete articulare genu, a network of small vessels proximal to and around the knee (Fig. 4).

The first, second, and third perforating branches, which in fact supply blood to the adductor muscles of the thigh, and a network of interconnecting branches of these vessels, which form a series of arcades, anastomose with the muscular branches of the PA and the genicular arteries. The termination of the DFA, sometimes called the fourth perforating artery, takes part in supplying blood to the network of muscular collateral vessels.

In the case of occlusion of the SFA, the blood is conducted to the PA by these two groups of vessels, which come together into the very well developed ramus muscularis, which runs in a transverse direction from the vastus medialis muscle to the PA. It is called by Martin the arteria collateralis magna (Martin et al. 1972; Fig. 4).

The profundapopliteal collateral circulation will be most effective if the PA and especially its proximal portion – the so-called collateral recipient segment – are free from arteriosclerotic lesions (Fig. 5a). There must be a free transition from the arteria collateralis magna into the PA.

If the occlusion of the SFA extends into the PA, the arteria collateralis magna is blocked and the collateral pathways will enter the PA more distally, making use of the medial and lateral superior genicular arteries and other vessels of the rete articulare genu, forming in this way profundapopliteal collaterals of the second category (Fig. 5b).

Further spread of the occlusion into the PA forces the collaterals to make use of branches of the more distally located middle genicular and sural arteries, the medial and lateral inferior genicular arteries, and small vessels of the rete patellae. These collaterals of the third category enter the PA at the level of the patella (Fig. 5c).

If the PA is totally occluded, collaterals of the fourth category, originating from the lateral and medial inferior genicular branches, enter the proximal parts of the anterior and posterior tibial arteries via anastomoses with the anterior and posterior recurrent tibial arteries (Fig. 5d).

The more distally the collaterals enter the main artery, the less is the capacity of the profundapopliteal collateral system.

The participation of the medial femoral circumflex artery in supplying the profundapopliteal collaterals is less important. This artery, in common with the ascending and transverse branches of the lateral femoral circumflex artery, acts more as a collector of

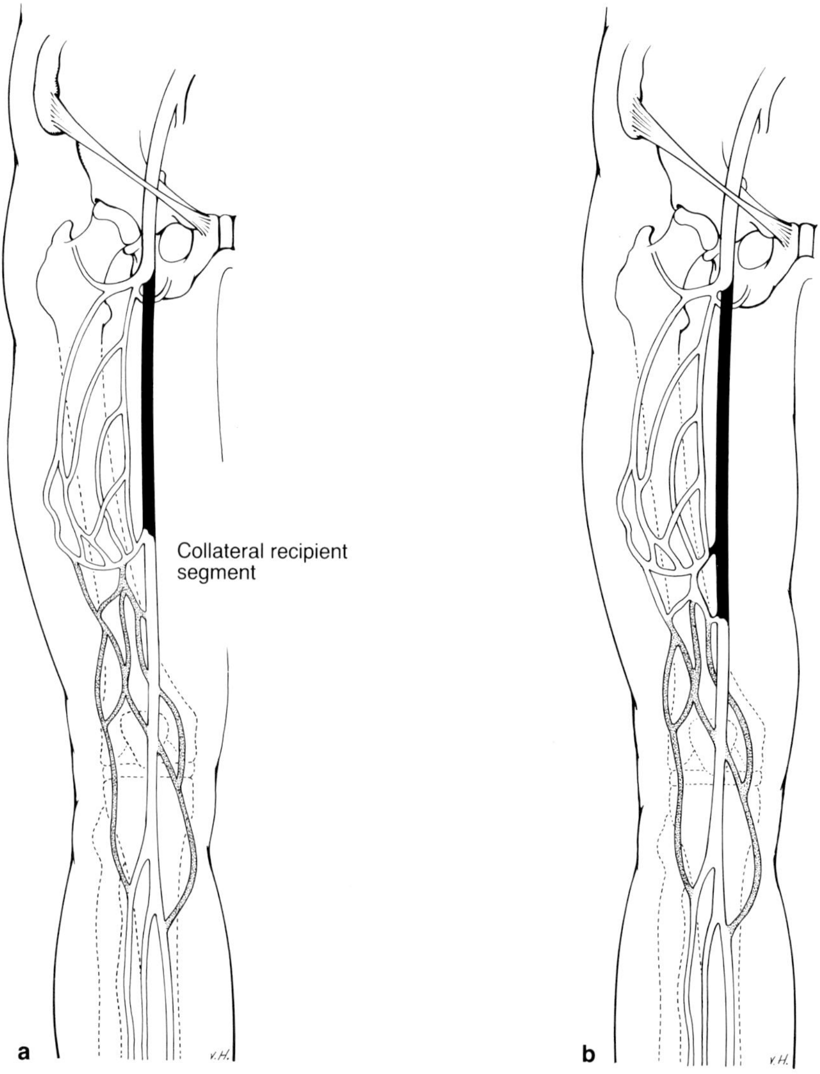

Fig. 5a–d. Four categories of femoropopliteal collaterals depending on the extent of the femoropopliteal arterial occlusion

blood originating from collaterals proximally, supplied by branches of the internal iliac artery (IIA; van Dongen 1957; Dietzek et al. 1990; Fig. 6). Collaterals provided by the obturator artery anastomose with the ascending and deep branches of the medial femoral circumflex artery, and collaterals furnished by the inferior gluteal artery anastomose with the superficial branch of the medial and with the transverse branch of the lateral femoral circumflex artery.

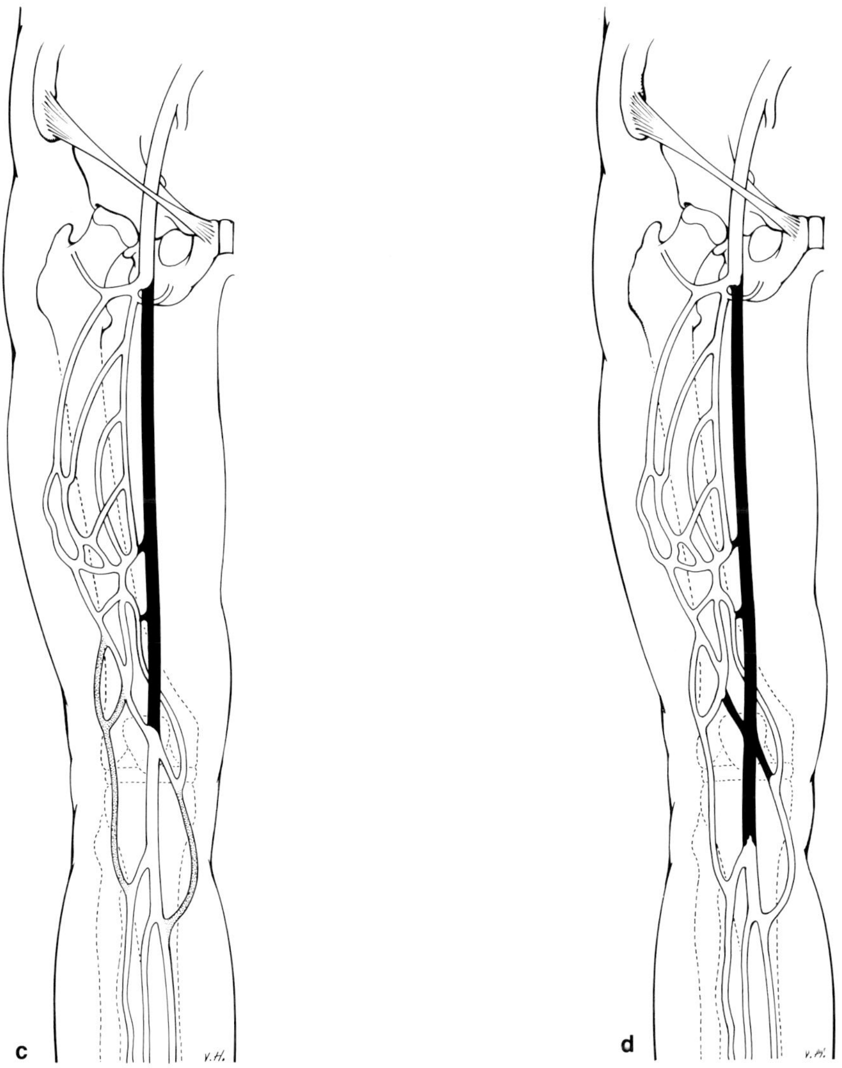

Fig. 5c–d

The ascending branch of the lateral femoral circumflex artery collects blood from collaterals provided by branches of the superior gluteal artery.

Collaterals between the lateral and medial femoral circumflex arteries and anastomoses with the first perforating (the cruciate anastomosis) form the connection between the branches of the IIA and the profundapopliteal collateral system. In this way an important chain of anastomoses extends from the pelvic arteries

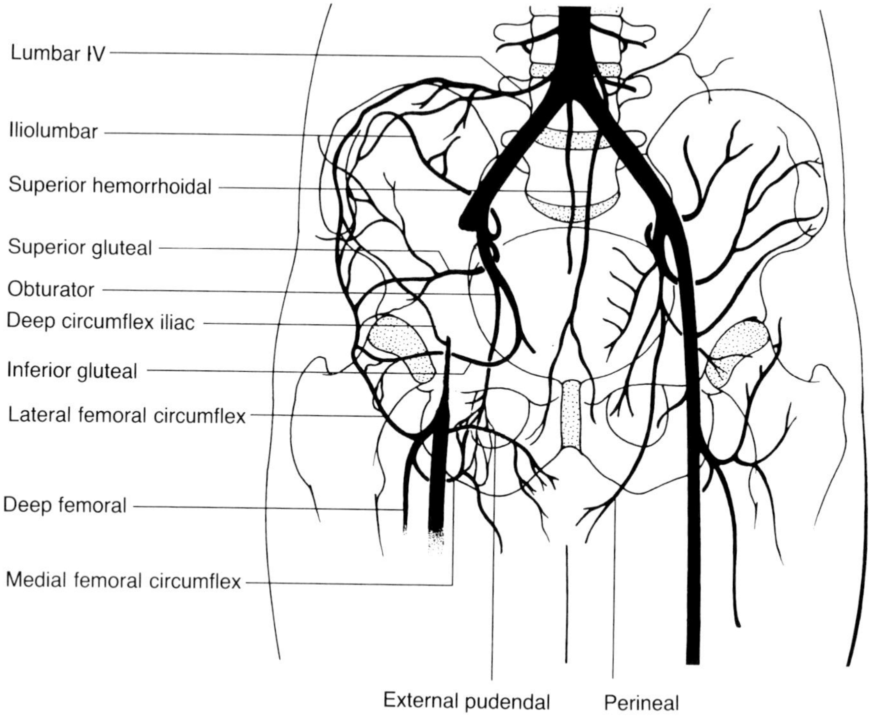

Fig. 6. Collateral circulation in occlusion of the external iliac artery (EIA) and the common femoral artery (CFA). Collaterals are supplied by the fourth lumbar artery, the right internal iliac artery (IIA) and its branches, and the superior hemorrhoidal artery. Retrograde filling of the medial and lateral femoral circumflex arteries takes place through these three groups of collaterals

proximally to the popliteal and tibial vessels distally. They form the morphologic basis for collateral blood flow in multilevel disease with varying degrees of obstruction in the iliac, common femoral, superficial femoral, and popliteal arteries.

References

Dietzek AM, Goldsmith J, Veith FJ, Sanchez LA, Gupta SK, Wengerter KR (1990) Interruption of critical aortoiliac collateral circulation during non-vascular operations: a cause of acute limb-threatening ischemia. J Vasc Surg 12: 645–653

King TA, DePalma RG, Rhodes RS (1984) Diabetes mellitus and atherosclerotic involvement of the profunda femoris artery. Surg Gynecol Obstet 159: 553–556

Martin P, Frawley JE, Barabas AP, Rosengarten DS (1972) On the surgery of atherosclerosis of the profunda femoris artery. Surgery 71: 182–189

Vaas F (1982) Atherosclerotic lesions at the bifurcation of the common femoral artery. Neth J Surg 34: 168–173

van Dongen RJAM (1957) Aortographic study of the collateral circulation in cases of occlusion of the aorta and pelvic arteries. Neth J Surg 9: 203–227

4 Clinical and Laboratory Investigations of the Obstruction of the Deep Femoral Artery

W.L. BRECKWOLDT and T.F. O'DONNELL JR

Considerable controversy has centered on the role of profundaplasty in vascular reconstruction. Few argue the benefits of profundaplasty when combined with an inflow procedure, but profundaplasty as the sole vascular procedure has been associated with mixed results, whether for claudication or limb salvage. Since the deep femoral artery (DFA) is involved in a high proportion of all patients undergoing arteriography for lower extremity ischemia – e.g., Beales et al. (1971) gives the figure 59% – the indications for profundaplasty must be addressed. The focus of this chapter will be: (a) the noninvasive preoperative evaluation of the DFA and predictors of success of profundaplasty and (b) noninvasive means of postoperative follow-up after profundaplasty.

Preoperative Evaluation of the Deep Femoral Artery

Clinical Examination

There are numerous techniques for detecting femoral popliteal occlusive disease, but few noninvasive means of isolating the effects of a diseased DFA. Patients with stenosis of the DFA can present with mild claudication to digital gangrene, depending upon the degree of coexistent vascular disease. Morris-Jones and Jones (1974) noted that in 55 patients with DFA stenosis combined with superficial femoral artery (SFA) occlusion, the majority (60%) presented with debilitating claudication alone, while 40% presented with ischemic rest pain or gangrene. Physical examination may reveal a femoral bruit or a diminished to absent femoral pulse. In their preoperative evaluation, Mitchell and coworkers (1979) detected normal femoral pulses in 20 out of 25 patients (80%) undergoing isolated profundaplasty. A femoral bruit was present in ten out of 25 (40%) of these patients.

Noninvasive Studies

Assessment of the DFA can be either hemodynamic or anatomical: hemodynamic methods include Doppler spectral analysis, Doppler systolic pressure (DSP), and pulse volume recording (PVR); anatomical methods include physical exmination, B-mode ultrasound, magnetic resonance imaging (MRI), and angiography. Most hemodynamic techniques indirectly determine the status of the DFA by process of elimination. While Doppler ultrasound determination of ankle-brachial indices (ABI) is useful in determining the functional state of limb perfusion, ABI are less reliable, even with segmental pressure measurements, in determining the anatomical location of vascular occlusive disease. A greater than 15 mmHg decrease in thigh pressure versus brachial pressure suggests aortoiliofemoral disease, but the thigh cuff pressure is also dependent upon the status of both the SFA and DFA. Further localization to the femoral segment and exclusion of iliac artery disease, therefore, must rely on physical examination (presence of normal femoral pulse), scrutiny of the femoral artery, continuous Doppler wave form, Doppler spectral analysis and its derivatives, or an additional "high thigh" cuff. Amplitude measurements of pulse volume recordings may offer a more objective assessment of the femoral pulse, but are subject to the same limitations encountered with segmental cuff pressures. A biphasic or triphasic femoral signal found on continuous wave Doppler examination of the femoral artery suggests adequate inflow and therefore significant femoral level disease if associated with a decreased thigh segmental Doppler pressure or PVR. Numerous techniques which derive hemodynamic formulas for detecting the presence of significant aortoiliac disease may rule out or confirm proximal inflow disease, but unfortunately cannot differentiate between occlusive disease of the SFA and DFA (O'Donnell et al. 1978).

B-mode ultrasound and duplex scanning are the mainstay of noninvasive evaluation of vascular disease (Jager et al. 1982; Strauss et al. 1991). B-mode ultrasound provides structural detail in terms of vessel lumen size and location of atherosclerotic disease. Spectral analysis in effect breaks down the Doppler signal into "velocity vectors." These vectors are then interpreted in terms of spectral height, a correlate of forward velocity, spectral width, a correlate of turbulent flow, and waveform contour, a correlate of vessel elasticity. Forward velocity increases with distal resistance, whether it be stenosis, vessel caliber, or anatomical resistance. At the site of a stenosis and the vessel just proximal to it, only a "jet" of flow crosses the narrowed vessel and flow velocity is at its greatest. Flow will decrease distal to a stenosis and proximal to an occlusion and will be reflected in the spectral height. Spectral width reflects turbulent flow across a vessel.

Turbulence and eddying currents increase and thus spectral broadening increases as the degree of stenosis increases. Spectral broadening also occurs at vessel bifurcations. The contour of the waveform – monophasic, biphasic, triphasic – correlates to vessel wall elasticity, i.e., whether the vessel has "rebound" following pulsatile flow. This rebound is detected as reverse flow (a negative spectral height) on spectral analysis. Atherosclerotic, stenotic arteries are rigid and lose their reverse flow (Fig. 1). Doppler color flow imaging, with its ease of displaying flow dynamics, provides a more "legible" image which can more easily reveal obstructions to flow and eddying currents (Fig. 2).

Thus spectral analysis and B-mode imaging provide information as to flow characteristics in addition to anatomy. Kohler et al. (1987) reported an 82% sensitivity and 92% specificity when utilizing duplex scanning to identify a greater than 50% reduction in the diameter of vessels of the lower extremity. Kohler reported, in 48 patients, a sensitivity of 67% and specificity of 81% when utilizing duplex imaging to detect a greater than 50% diameter reduction in the DFA alone. A 53% positive predictive value and an 88% negative predictive value were then calculated for this imaging modality versus angiography. Strauss et al. (1991) studied the use of duplex scanning of DFA stenosis of more than 30% in diameter (50% of area) by measuring both peak systolic and time-averaged maximal flow. They found (in 123 examinations) a sensitivity of 91% and 96% and a specificity of 85% and 98%. The positive predictive values were 86% and 98% and the negative predictive values 91% and 96% (all values respectively for a peak systolic velocity of 180 cm/s and more or for a time-averaged maximal velocity of 50 cm/s). Furthermore, both of these measures were highly reproducible on a day to day basis in the same patient. The lower predictive values for the DFA versus other vessels of the lower extremity probably relates to the depth of the DFA in the thigh.

MRI as a noninvasive means of evaluating the peripheral vascular tree has shown promise, but its development is still in progress (Wedeen et al. 1985; Steinberg et al. 1990). Although MRI has improved over the past 5 years, evaluation of flow characteristics and hemodynamics has been difficult due to flow artifact and variations in flow velocity during the cardiac cycle. MRI has been especially difficult in the lower extremity due to overlapping anatomy in a two-plane projection: with the current status of MR

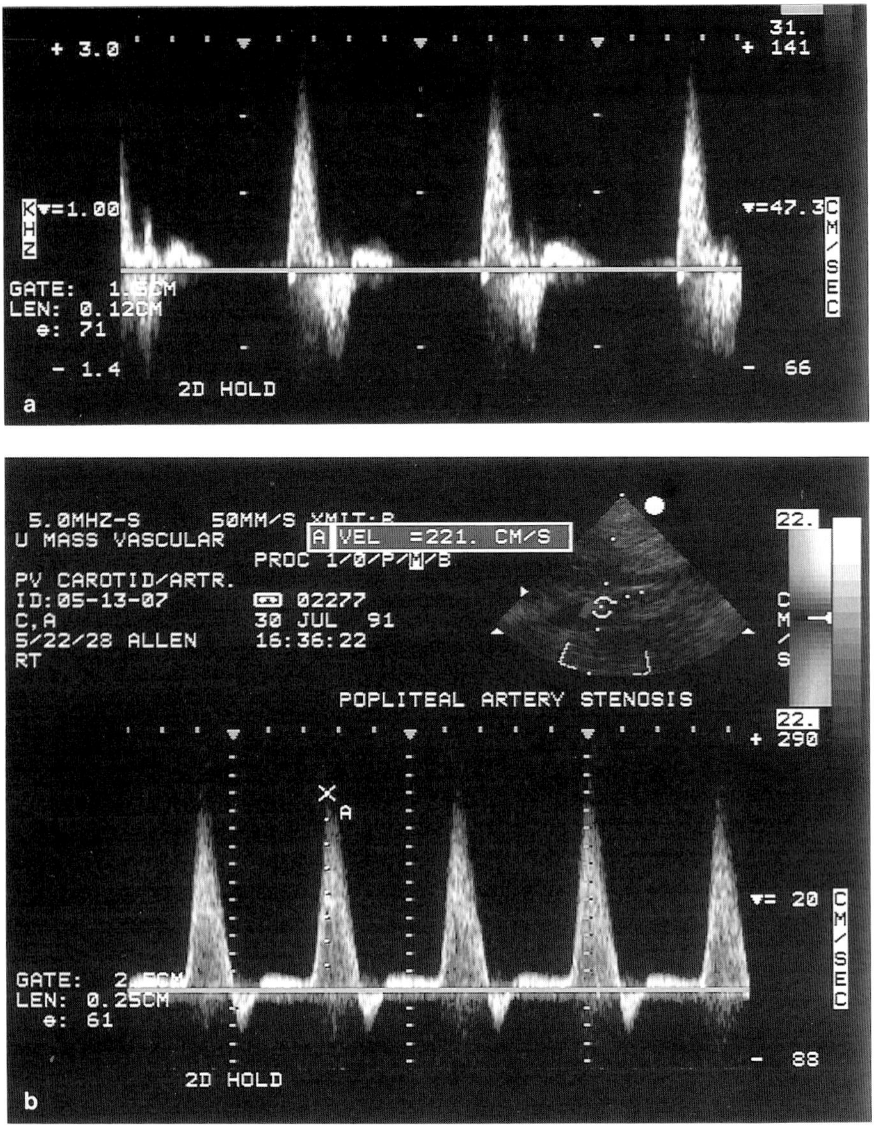

Fig. 1. **a** Spectral analysis of a normal artery. Note normal spectral height and width. Triphasic contour. **b** Spectral analysis of vessel with high-grade stenosis. Spectral height is increased and spectral broadening is evident. **c** Spectral analysis of vessel distal to high-grade stenosis. Spectral height is decreased and width nears normal. Triphasic signal returns

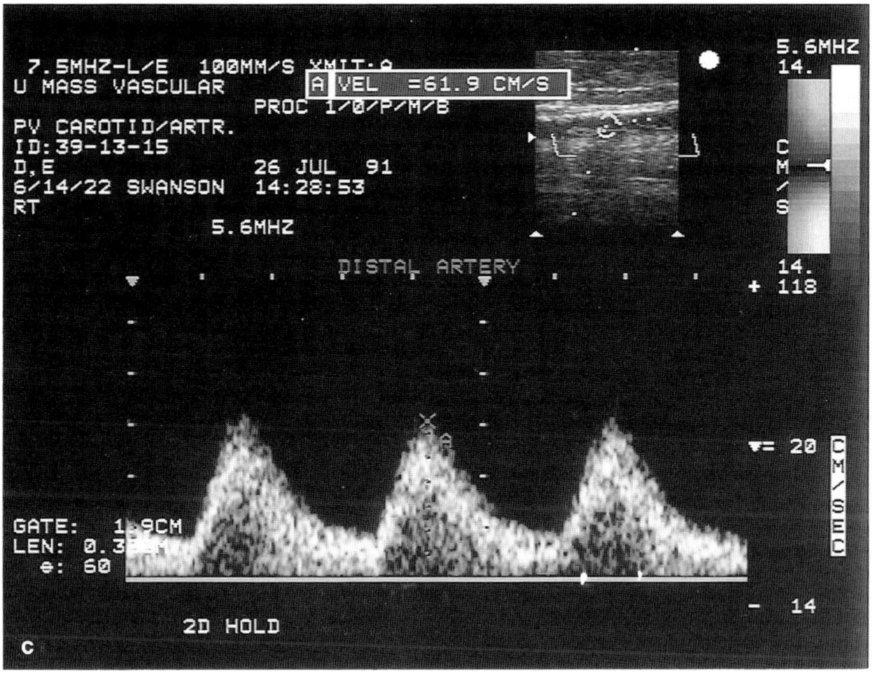

Fig. 1c

resolution in the lower extremity, standard invasive angiography is still the gold standard. The cost of routine MRI at the time of writing is prohibitive and reserved for special cases. Its role in evaluating the DFA is yet to be determined.

Noninvasive Predictors of Success of Profundaplasty

Relief or improvement of symptoms in isolated DFA revascularization has been reported to be 20%–100% in patients with claudication and 45%–90% in patients with critical ischemia (Leather et al. 1978; Boren et al. 1980; Fernandes e Fernandes et al. 1978; Ward and Morris-Jones 1977). Once a stenosis of the DFA has been established by angiography or duplex scanning, the surgeon must determine whether profundaplasty alone will benefit the patient.

Mitchell et al. (1979) evaluated the clinical correlates of success of profundaplasty. Sixty percent of patients with a preoperatively decreased femoral pulse had successful improvement of symptoms, whereas those with a normal preoperative femoral pulse had a

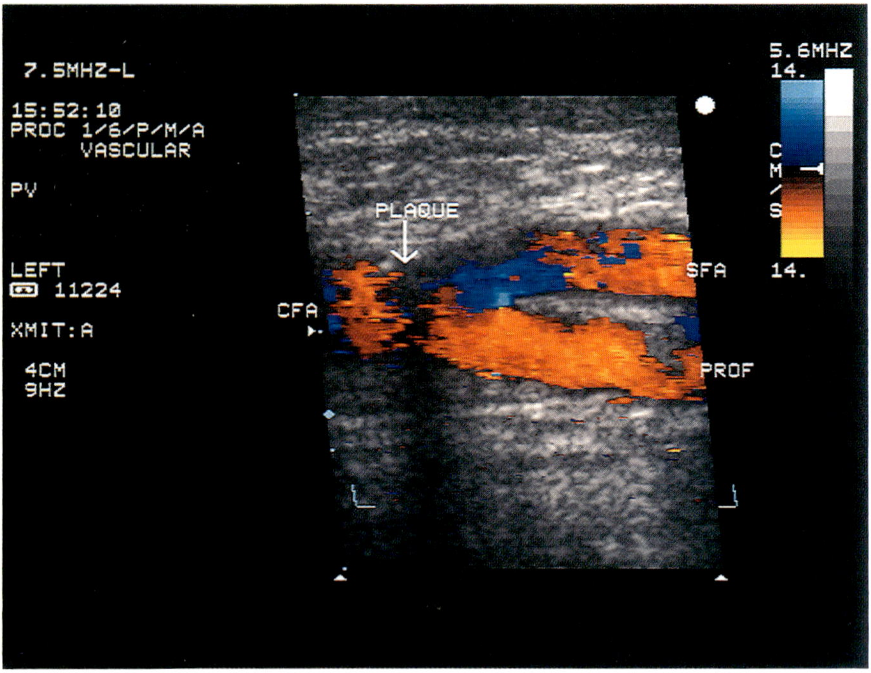

Fig. 2. Duplex scan of deep femoral artery (DFA, *PROF*) with color enhancement. Note atherosclerotic plaque (*arrow*) at bifurcation but otherwise normal profunda. *SFA*, superficial femoral artery; *CFA*, common femoral artery. The *red* images signify flow away from the heart (*left* to *right*) and the *blue* images toward the heart (*right* to *left*)

45% success rate. Seventy percent of patients with a preoperative femoral bruit had improvement of symptoms, while 30% of those without bruit improved with profundaplasty alone. While Mitchell's results were not significant, his findings do suggest that presence of a decreased femoral pulse or femoral bruit may be a predictor of success of profundaplasty.

Simple ankle pressure indices and ABI have not been shown to be predictive of a successful profundaplasty. Determination of the collateral flow across the popliteal segment using Doppler pressure has been reported by Boren et al. to predict success of isolated profundaplasty. This calculation, the profundapopliteal collateral index (PPCI), is determined from the following equation:

$$\frac{(AK - BK)}{AK}$$

where AK is above-knee doppler pressure and BK is below-knee doppler pressure. Boren et al. (1980) noted in their series that if the PPCI was <0.25, limb salvage was achieved in 67% of patients with critical ischemia. If the PPCI was >0.50, profundaplasty did not succeed. Ouriel et al. (1987) confirmed the utility of the PPCI in patients undergoing profundaplasty in conjunction with an inflow procedure: for a PPCI >0.25, 20% success in symptom relief was noted, and for PPCI <0.25, 85% of patients noted symptomatic improvement.

In a prospective study of Doppler pressures and segmental plethysmographic amplitude in patients before and after aorto-femoral bypass, we (O'Donnell et al. 1979) evaluated various predictive indices derived from these hemodynamic measurements.

We examined predictive hemodynamic calculations for determining success of inflow procedures combined with profundaplasty in patients with combined aortoiliac and femoral popliteal (AIFP) occlusive disease. The thigh to arm DSP ratio, an index of inflow disease, was comparable between the AIFP disease success (0.55 ± 0.1) and AIFP failure (0.61 ± 0.7) groups. This finding indicates that adequate flow had been restored to thigh level in both groups. Derivatives of the segmental DSP such as the thigh–ankle, thigh–calf, and calf–ankle measurements showed no statistically significant difference between success and failure groups when compared to brachial pressures. Our findings are in contrast to those of Boren and associates (1980). On the other hand, one of the PVR indices did have predictive value. This calculation, designated the FPΩ index, was significantly lower in the AIFP success groups (0.048 ± 0.06) than in the failure groups (0.13 ± 0.6) when subjected to chi-squared analysis. The FPΩ is calculated as follows:

$$\frac{\text{thigh PVR} - \text{ankle PVR}}{15}$$

where 15 represents the arm, or normal PVR. An FPΩ index of <0.2 was associated with successful results in all 11 limbs in the success group, but was also found in five limbs of the failure group. In contrast, the remaining six limbs in the failure group had an FPΩ >0.2. It would appear that the FPΩ index has a high degree of accuracy in predicting failure in patients with combined segment disease and approximately a 2:3 chance of predicting success. The ability to preoperatively determine which limb will be both clinically and functionally improved after an inflow procedure combined with profundaplasty has significant value. Much value has been placed on the patency of the popliteal artery and runoff potential, as in the PPCI, but, in our blinded assessment of the success and failure groups undergoing combined procedures (O'Donnell et al. 1979), the incidence of patency of the popliteal artery and its runoff were comparable between groups. Derivatives of the DSP reflect the resistance to blood flow across that particular segment (Sumner and Strandness 1978). Segmental plethysmography may more closely reflect total volume of blood flow under the monitoring cuff as its measurement is dependent upon the number of vessels, whether they be segmental or collateral vessels, surrounded by the monitoring cuff and not the occlusion pressure of one single vessel. The FPΩ index may better represent the potential recipient vascular bed of the DFA and its collateral supply to the ankle: the PPCI represents the collateral circulation at the popliteal level only. Indeed, in our combined segment limbs, a FPΩ value of greater than 0.2 had a high probability of failure.

When using the aforementioned formulas, one must keep in mind that both the FPΩ and PPCI are derived calculations. The PPCI reflects popliteal collateral flow, while the FPΩ reflects popliteal collateral flow and runoff. Neither calculation has a substantial predictive value (<85% at best), but both are more effective at predictive failure (80%–100%). Such calculations should not preclude further noninvasive and/or invasive testing of the vascular anatomy. In other words, the vascular surgeon should not rely solely on the PPCI or FPΩ in determining need for profundaplasty alone or in conjunction with another vascular procedure.

The utility of duplex scanning, color flow Doppler imaging, and MR angiography as predictors of profundaplasty success has not been determined. Certain angiographic criteria that predict success may be extrapolated to these noninvasive modalities, as the information gained from these studies is similar. These criteria include popliteal artery patency, two- to three-vessel runoff, and DFA patency. Ouriel et al. (1987) noted that 37 out of 41 patients (90%) undergoing profundaplasty combined with an inflow procedure who had a patent popliteal segment had a successful result. Of ten patients with an occluded popliteal segment, only three (30%) had a successful result. Mitchell et al. (1979) reported a 67% success rate in patients undergoing isolated profundaplasty with a patent popliteal artery versus a 17% success rate in those with an occluded popliteal. Morris-Jones and Jones (1974) noted a decline in success of profundaplasty as the number of patent runoff vessels declined. For instance, success was best achieved with three-vessel runoff and the poorest results were obtained with zero- to one-vessel runoff. Mitchell et al. (1979) noted a 0% profundaplasty success rate in patients who had disease of the distal DFA. One must note that these studies were performed utilizing angiography, but the same information can be obtained from the noninvasive modalities as mentioned.

Means of Profundaplasty Follow-Up

The most important means of follow-up after profundaplasty is clearly clinical status. Limb loss, need for distal reconstruction, unimproved or worsening claudication signify treatment failure. Loss of femoral pulse or femoral occlusion by the aforementioned imaging techniques also imply DFA occlusion.

Changes in ABI following profundaplasty are variable (Table 1). Several authors note no change in ABI following profundaplasty (Ward and Morris-Jones 1977; Wright 1983), but others note significant improvement in both isolated profundaplasties (Hansen et al. 1990; Jamil et al. 1984) and those performed in conjunction with an inflow procedure (Ouriel et al. 1987). It appears that improvement of ABI in a series correlates with the success rate of that series: in other words, patient selection and indications for profundaplasty may vary between groups. Jamil et al. (1984) noted that in their "clinically successful" profundaplasties, mean postoperative ABI were nearly double that of preoperative values, whereas in the clinical failure group there was no change between pre- and postoperative ABI. Although ABI have no predictive value, an improvement of ABI postoperatively does roughly correlate with success of profundaplasty.

Exercise tolerance testing and reactive hyperemia are probably more sensitive indicators of profundaplasty success and better correlates of symptomatic improvement. Fernandes e Fernandes et al. (1978) noted that in 20 patients undergoing profundaplasty for severe claudication, 80% showed improvement in ABI. One hundred percent showed improvement in walking distance on treadmill testing and in postexercise ankle pressure. Wright (1983) noted that in 15 patients studies, there were no postoperative changes in resting calf muscle blood flow, as measured by xenon-133 clearance studies and by venous occlusion plethysmography.

Table 1. Changes in ankle-brachial indices (ABI) following profundaplasty

Author	Patients (*n*)	Change in ABI
Ward and Morris-Jones (1977)	12	−0.02
Wright (1983)	15	+0.02
Hansen et al. (1990)	21	+0.15
Rollins et al. (1985)	56	+0.08
Jamil et al. (1984)	88	+0.24 (successes) +0.06 (failures)

Significant ($p < 0.01$) increases in maximal blood flow were detected 1 min after maximal exercise, and significant ($p < 0.01$) acceleration of reactive hyperemia in the calf was noted as well. The work of Jamil et al. (1980) using venous occlusion plethysmography confirms these results.

No studies have been performed using duplex scanning for follow-up after profundaplasty and this is probably not cost-effective.

References

Beales JS, Adcock FA, Frawley JS et al (1971) The radiological assessment of disease of the profunda femoris artery. Br J Radiol 44: 854–859

Boren CH, Towne JB, Bernhard VM, Salles-Cunha S (1980) Profundapopliteal collateral index. A guide to successful profundaplasty. Arch Surg 115: 1366–1372

Fernandes e Fernandes J, Nicolaides AN, Angelides NA, Gordon-Smith IC (1978) An objective assessment of common femoral endarterectomy and profundaplasty in patients with superficial femoral occlusion. Surgery 83: 313–318

Hansen AK, Bille S, Nielsen PH, Egeblad K (1990) Profundaplasty as the only reconstructive procedure in patients with severe ischemia of the lower extremity. Surg Gynecol Obstet 171: 47–50

Jager KA, Ricketts HJ, Strandness D (1982) Duplex scanning for the evaluation of lower limb arterial disease. In: Bernstein EF, Barnes RB (eds) Noninvasive diagnostic techniques in vascular disease. Mosby, St Louis, pp 619–631

Jamil Z, Hobson RW, Mehta K, O'Donnell TF Jr, Jain K, Lee BC (1980) Alterations in calf blood flow following profundaplasty. J Surg Res 28: 230–234

Jamil Z, Hobson RW, Lynch TG et al (1984) Revascularization of the profunda femoris artery for limb salvage. Am Surg 50: 109–111

Kohler TR, Nance DR, Cramer MM, Vandenburghe N, Strandness DE Jr (1987) Duplex scanning for diagnosis of aortoiliac and femoropopliteal disease: a prospective study. Circulation 76: 1074–1080

Leather RP, Shah DM, Karmody AM (1978) The use of extended profundaplasty in limb salvage. Am J Surg 136: 359–362

Mitchell RA, Bone GE, Bridges R, Pomajzi MJ, Fry WJ (1979) Patient selection for isolated profundaplasty. Arteriographic correlates of operative results. Am J Surg 138: 912–919

Morris-Jones W, Jones CD (1974) Profundaplasty in the treatment of femoropopliteal occlusion. Am J Surg 127: 680–686

O'Donnell TF Jr, Cossman D, Callow AD (1978) Noninvasive intraoperative monitoring: a prospective study comparing Doppler systolic occlusion pressure and segmental plethysmography. Am J Surg 135: 539–546

O'Donnell TF Jr, Lahey SJ, Kelly JJ, Ransil BJ, Millan VG et al (1979) A prospective study of Doppler pressures and segmental plethysmography before and following aortofemoral bypass. Implications for predicting success and for adopting a uniform method of classifying arterial disease. Surgery 86: 120–129

Ouriel K, DeWeese JA, Ricotta JJ, Green RM (1987) Revascularization of the distal profunda femoris artery in the reconstructive treatment of aortoiliac occlusive disease. J Vasc Surg 6: 217–220

Rollins DL, Towne JB, Bernhard VM, Baum PL (1985) Isolated profundaplasty for limb salvage. J Vasc Surg 2: 585–590

Sumner DS, Strandness DE (1978) Aortoiliac reconstruction in patients with combined iliac and superficial femoral artery occlusion. Surgery 84: 348–355

Steinberg FL, Yucel EK, Dumoulin CL, Souza SP (1990) Peripheral vascular and abdominal applications of MR flow imaging techniques. Magn Reson Med 14: 315–320

Strauss AL, Schäberle W, Rieger H, Roth FJ (1991) Use of duplex scanning in the diagnosis of arteria profunda femoris stenosis. J Vasc Surg 13: 698–704

Ward AS, Morris-Jones W (1977) The long term results of profundaplasty in femoropopliteal arterial occlusion. Br J Surg 64: 365–367

Wedeen VJ, Meuli RA, Edelman RR et al (1985) Projective imaging of pulsatile flow with magnetic resonance. Science 230: 946–948

Wright CJ (1983) Effect of femoral profundaplasty on blood flow. Can J Surg 26: 325–327

5 Roentgenologic Aspects of the Obstruction of the Deep Femoral Artery

E.V. KINNEY and J.B. TOWNE

The deep femoral artery (DFA) is the primary source of blood flow to the thigh and the major collateral source for the leg when the superficial femoral artery (SFA) is occluded (Towne and Rollins 1986). With increased recognition of the importance of the DFA as a collateral vessel in atherosclerotic peripheral vascular disease, improved techniques for arteriographic visualization of the DFA have been developed, allowing classification based on atherosclerotic disease distribution. Specific roentgenographic patterns of atherosclerotic disease can then be correlated with the results of surgical revascularization of the DFA.

In this chapter we will review: normal roentgenographic appearance of the DFA, its branches, and collateral connections; radiologic techniques important for optimal visualization of the DFA; patterns of atherosclerotic disease of the DFA; and the relation of atherosclerotic disease distribution to successful revascularization of the DFA.

Normal Anatomy

The DFA usually arises from the posterolateral aspect of the common femoral artery (CFA) 3–5 cm below the inguinal ligament; it takes a lateral or posterolateral course to the SFA in 48% of cases and a directly posterior course to the SFA in 40% (Fig. 1). In 10% of cases the DFA runs medial to the SFA, and in 2% large branches of the DFA are found both medial and lateral to the SFA.

The branching pattern is variable. In 58% the DFA gives rise to both the medial and lateral circumflex vessels, in 18% the medial femoral circumflex is a direct branch of the CFA, and in 15% the lateral femoral circumflex is a direct branch of the CFA (Fig. 2). When the lateral femoral circumflex arises directly from the CFA, the main trunk of the DFA takes a medial or

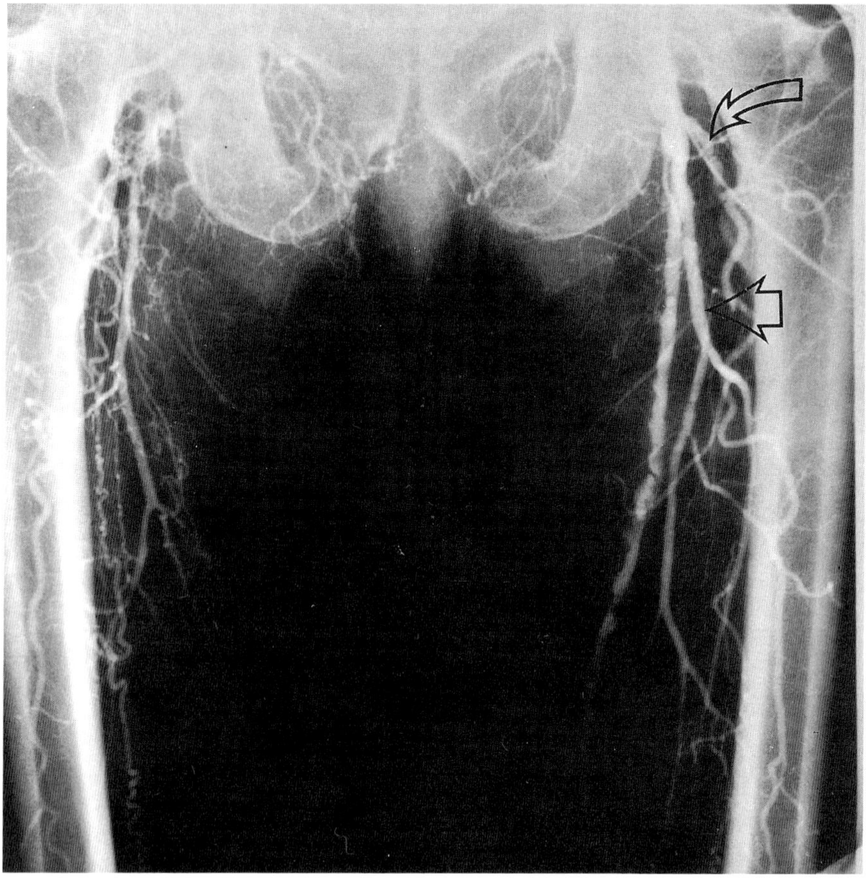

Fig. 1. Normal anatomy: deep femoral artery (DFA) usually takes a lateral or posterolateral course to the superior femoral artery (SFA). Main trunk of DFA (*straight arrow*) and lateral femoral circumflex branch of DFA (*curved arrow*) are shown. On the right, note complete sparing of the DFA system despite common femoral artery (CFA) and SFA occlusion

posteromedial course to the SFA. The main trunk of the DFA passes inferiorly, just medial to the femur, and gives off three perforating branches. The terminal portion of the DFA, sometimes referred to as the fourth perforating branch, makes connection to the highest genicular branch of the popliteal artery (PA) in the area of the adductor hiatus (Fig. 3).

The lateral femoral circumflex passes transversely and divides into ascending, transverse, and descending branches. The ascending branch passes upward to the lateral aspect of the hip, there making connection with branches of the inferior gluteal artery. The

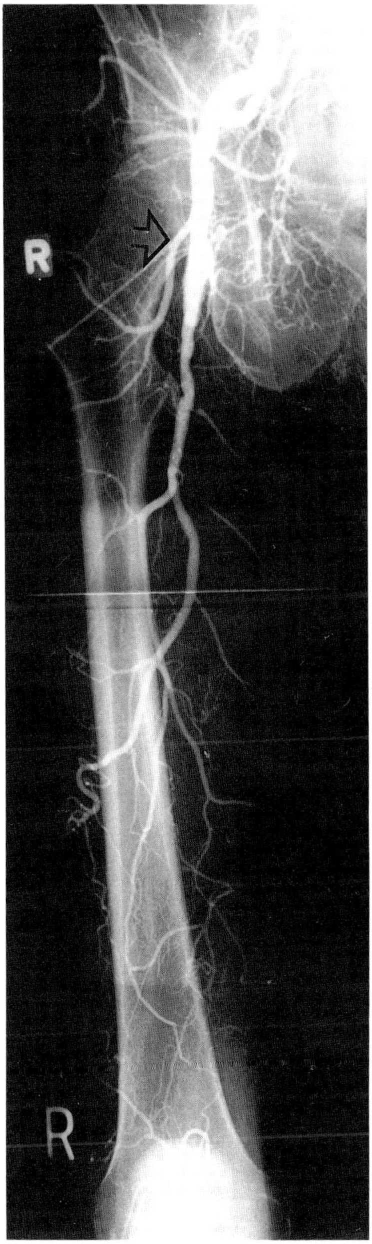

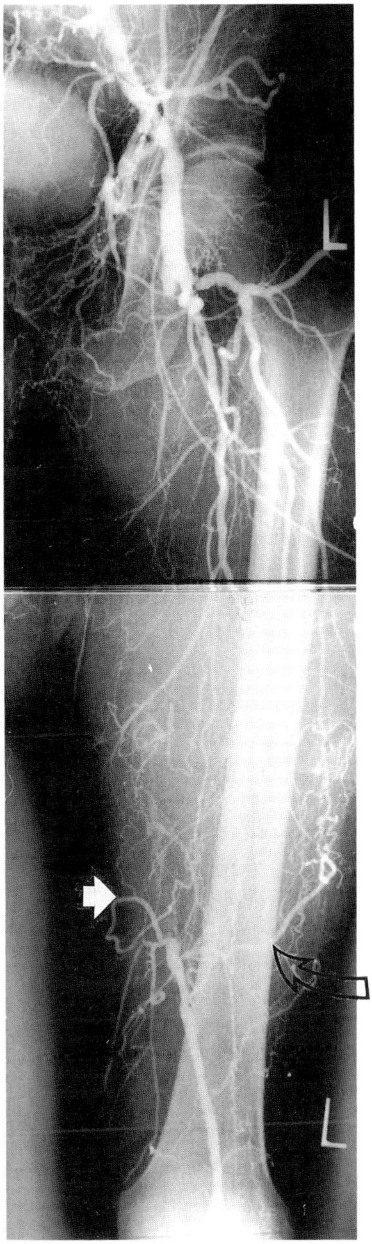

Fig. 2

Fig. 3

Fig. 2. Anatomical variant. In 15% of cases, the lateral femoral circumflex is a direct branch of the common femoral artery (CFA; *arrow*)

Fig. 3. Normal deep femoral artery (DFA) collateral system with superficial femoral artery (SFA) occlusion. Note collateral connections between the descending branch of the lateral femoral circumflex and the lateral superior genicular branch of the popliteal artery (PA, *curved arrow*). Also note collateral connections between the terminal branches of the DFA and the highest genicular artery (*straight arrow*)

descending branch passes inferiorly, lateral to the femur to the level of the knee, where it makes connection with the lateral superior genicular branch of the popliteal artery (Fig. 3). The medial femoral circumflex passes posteromedial to the area of the obturator foramen, where it makes connection to branches of the obturator artery.

Collateral Pathways

When the CFA, SFA, or PA is involved with atherosclerotic disease, the DFA and its collateral connections become the major source of blood supply to the leg and foot. In cases of SFA occlusion, the descending branch of the lateral femoral circumflex and the third and fourth perforating branches are the major collaterals (Haimovici et al. 1960) (Fig. 4). The most important genicular branches are the highest genicular and the lateral superior genicular arteries. When the CFA is occluded, collateral connections between the obturator and inferior gluteal arteries and the medial and lateral femoral circumflex arteries transport blood from the internal iliac artery (IIA) to the DFA (Margulis et al. 1957) (Fig. 5). In cases of combined SFA and PA occlusion, the DFA connects to the tibial vessels via the highest genicular artery with its musculoarticular and saphenous branches, the fourth perforating branch and descending branch of the lateral femoral circumflex, the genicular collateral network around the knee, and the recurrent tibial arteries (Fig. 6).

Angiographic Techniques

Angiographic demonstration of atherosclerotic disease of the DFA has improved with the advent of new and better techniques and the addition of lateral and oblique views to the standard anteroposterior projection. The most frequent site of atherosclerotic involvement of the DFA is near its origin. Disease at this level may not be apparent on frontal views, because the DFA usually arises from the posterolateral aspect of the CFA. In this view, the proximal portion of the vessel is foreshortened and often obscured. In a series of 209 lower extremity angiograms in which frontal, lateral, and oblique views were performed, Beales et al. (1971) demonstrated >50% stenosis of the DFA orifice in 9.5%. In 67.9% the stenotic segment was recognized only on the oblique or lateral

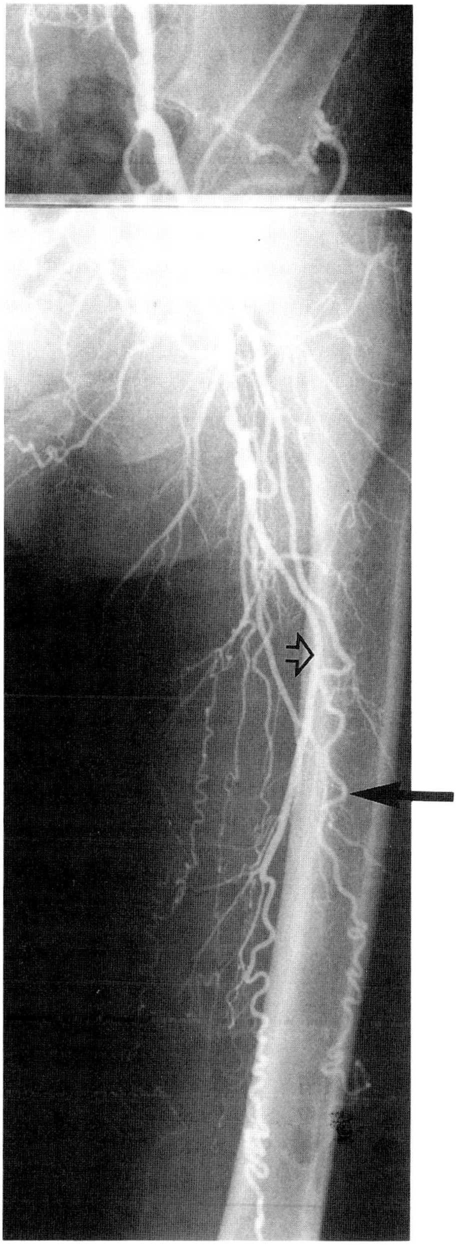

Fig. 4.

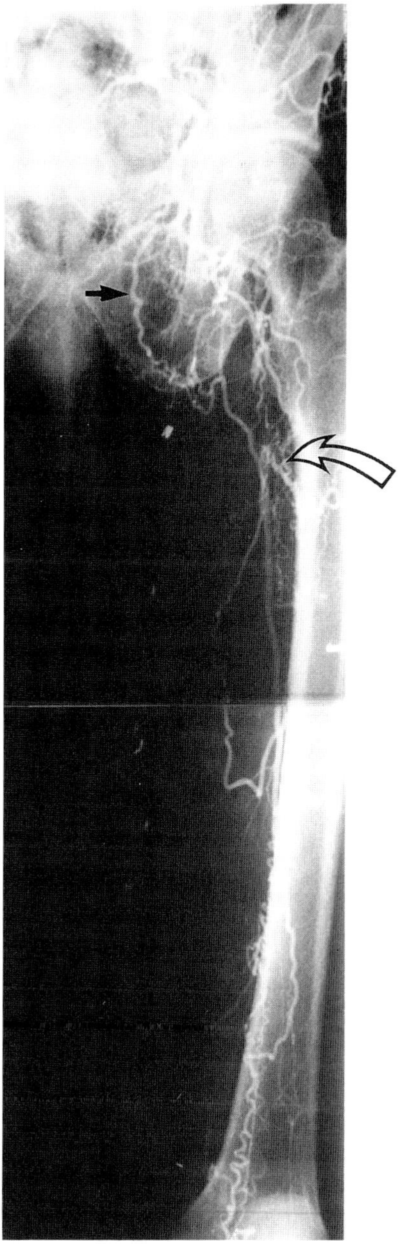

Fig. 5.

Fig. 4. Important collateral pathways. Descending branch of lateral femoral circumflex (*solid arrow*) and terminal portion of main deep femoral artery (DFA) trunk (*hollow arrow*) are shown

Fig. 5. Collateral pathways (*solid arrow*) between the internal iliac artery (IIA) and the deep femoral artery (DFA) reconstitute the main trunk of the DFA at the level of the first muscular perforating branch (*curved arrow*). In this case the external iliac artery (EIA), the common femoral artery (CFA), and the superficial femoral artery (SFA) are occluded

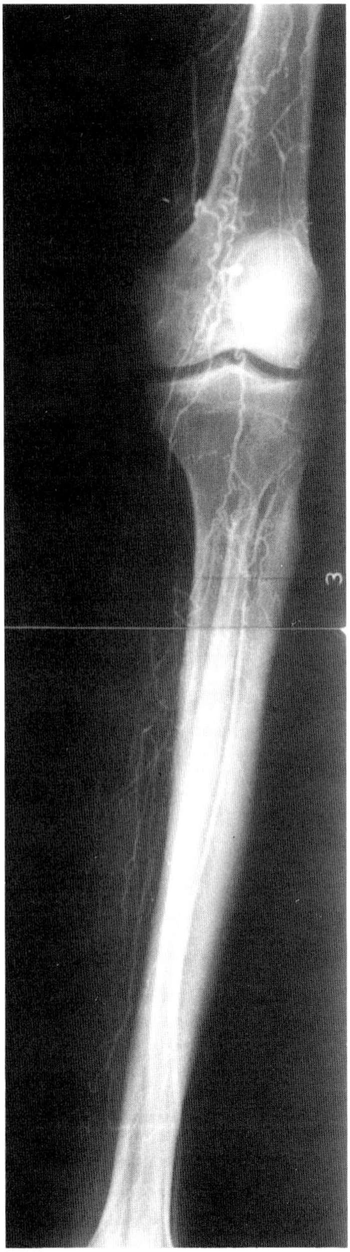

Fig. 6. Collateral pathways. In this case of combined superficial femoral artery (SFA) and popliteal artery (PA) occlusion, distal branches of the deep femoral artery (DFA) reconstitute the anterior tibial artery via the genicular collateral network and the recurrent tibial arteries

views, clearly showing the necessity of oblique views for adequate roentgenographic assessment (Fig. 7a,b). All of our patients with atherosclerotic occlusive disease are examined via the Seldinger technique, usually from a common femoral approach. If the common femoral approach is not feasible, access is obtained via the axillary artery. Digital subtraction, image intensification, and magnification are then used to obtain anteroposterior, right anterior oblique, and left anterior oblique views of the iliac and femoral arteries. Arterial runoff below the femoral bifurcation is assessed using sequential anteroposterior cut films. If the crural and/or pedal runoff is particularly sluggish, cut films may not allow adequate visualization. When the cut films of the tibial vessels are inadequate, digital subtraction, magnification, and multiple views are used to facilitate complete assessment.

In patients with mild to moderate renal failure in whom contrast volume is of concern, intra-arterial digital techniques are used to obtain the oblique view, which uses a minimum of contrast material. If these patients are well hydrated prior to the angiogram and if brisk diuresis is obtained during the contrast injection, there usually are no renal problems with this technique.

Roentgenographic Patterns of Disease

Among patients with atherosclerotic occlusive disease of the lower extremity, the DFA is frequently found to be disease free. Haimovici (1967), in a series of 321 arteriograms, found atherosclerotic involvement of the DFA in 9.5% of nondiabetics and 30.5% of diabetic patients. Similarly, Margulis et al. (1957) noted significant atherosclerotic involvement of the DFA in 18% of 168 limbs (Fig. 8).

When the DFA is involved with atherosclerosis, it is almost never the only vessel affected. Haimovici (1967) found significant DFA involvement in 5.8% of limbs with a femoral–popliteal pattern of atherosclerotic disease, 14% of limbs with femoral–popliteal–tibial disease, and 17.9% of limbs with combined aortoiliac and femoral–popliteal disease. Among limbs with superficial femoral artery occlusion, Beales et al. (1971) found 50% diameter-reducing orificial stenosis of the DFA in 14 of 114 cases (12%).

When the proximal DFA is affected by significant atherosclerosis, complete occlusion is uncommon, ranging from 0% to 4%. Atherosclerotic involvement of the distal DFA or its branches is considerably less common than proximal of orificial DFA stenosis. Martin et al. (1972) found that atherosclerotic involvement of the DFA was restricted to the segment from the orifice to the first perforator in 74% (Fig. 9) and was localized to the orifice

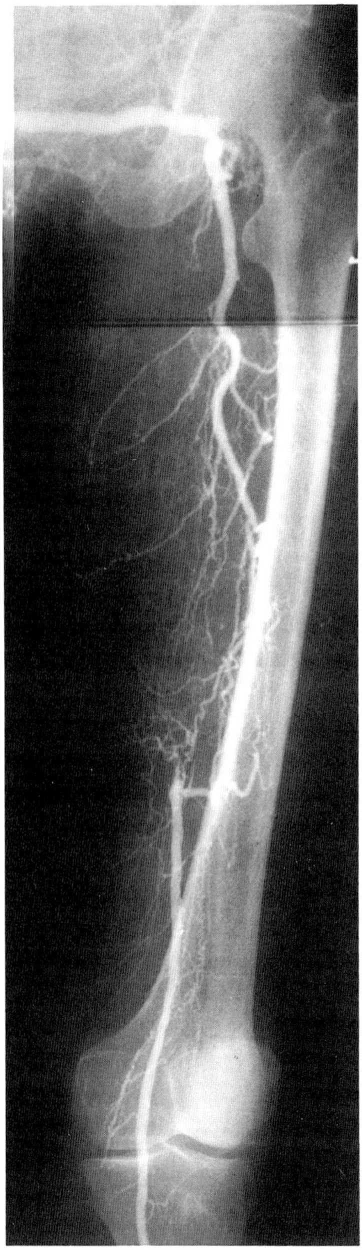

Fig. 7a

Fig. 7. a Anteroposterior cut film of femoral–femoral bypass. **b** Left anterior oblique view of femoral–femoral bypass using digital subtraction and magnification reveals a high-grade stenosis of the proximal deep femoral artery (DFA) that was not apparent on the standard anteroposterior cut film

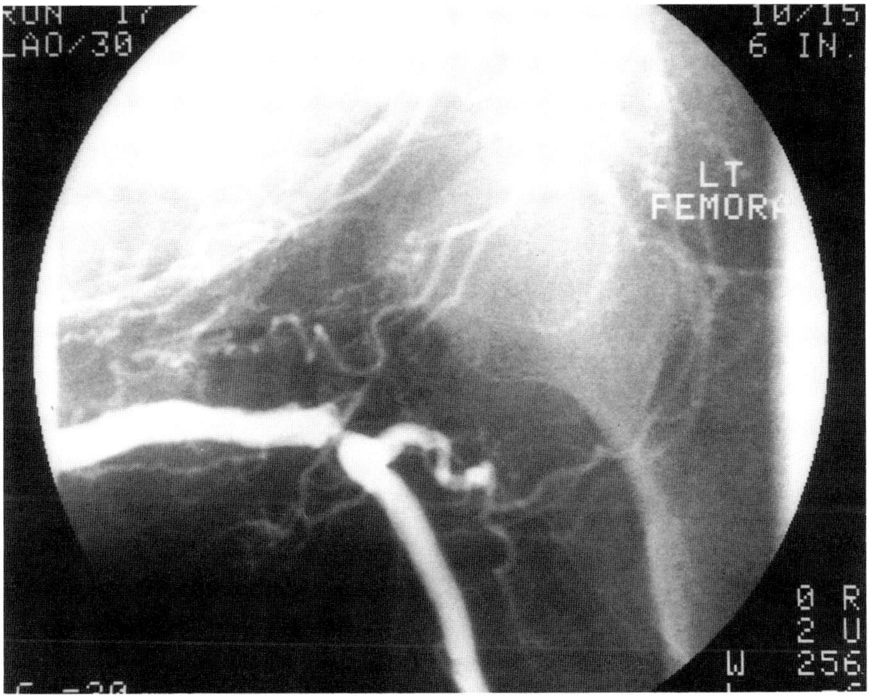

Fig. 7b

alone in 55% of cases (Fig. 10). In 12% of DFA affected by atherosclerosis, disease was located between the first perforating artery and the terminal segment. Diffuse involvement of the DFA was seen in 14% (Fig. 11). Similarly, Thompson et al. (1976) found atherosclerotic disease of the DFA to be confined to the proximal segment in 76% of cases and be orificial in 62%.

Arteriographic Correlations with the Results of Deep Femoral Artery Revascularization

Roentgenographic assessment of the severity and distribution of atherosclerotic disease is the usual starting point for planning revascularization. Early attempts to correlate specific roentgenographic patterns of atherosclerotic disease with the results of DFA revascularization were hindered by a lack of objective assessment. While several early reports suggested that profundaplasty could be beneficial in all patients with critical ischemia, irrespective of the distribution of atherosclerotic disease, later more careful studies have defined those specific situations in which DFA revascularization will predictably relieve ischemia.

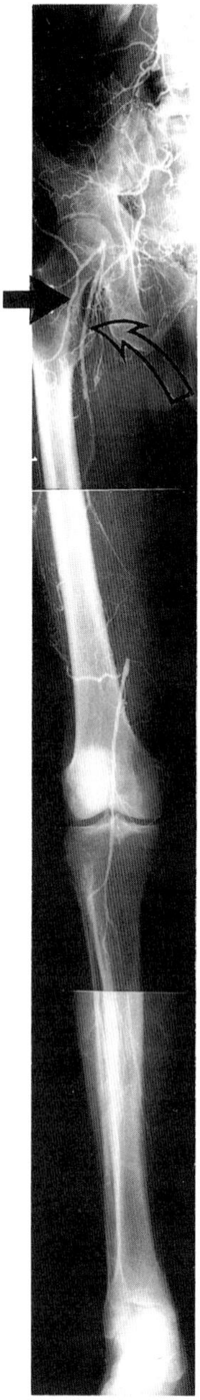

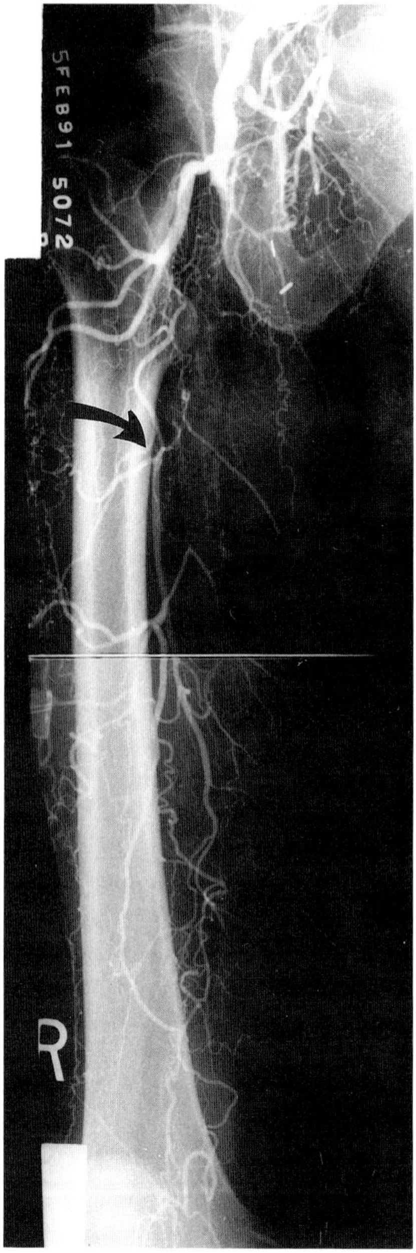

Fig. 8 **Fig. 9**

Fig. 8. Patterns of disease. Among patients with atherosclerotic occlusive disease, the deep femoral artery (DFA) is frequently disease free. In this case of iliac, common femoral (CFA), and superficial femoral (SFA) artery occlusion, the DFA system is intact. Descending branch of lateral femoral circumflex (*solid arrow*) and main DFA trunk (*curved arrow*) are shown

Fig. 9. Patterns of disease. Proximal deep femoral artery (DFA) occlusion with reconstitution of the main DFA trunk at the level of the first muscular perforating artery (*arrow*)

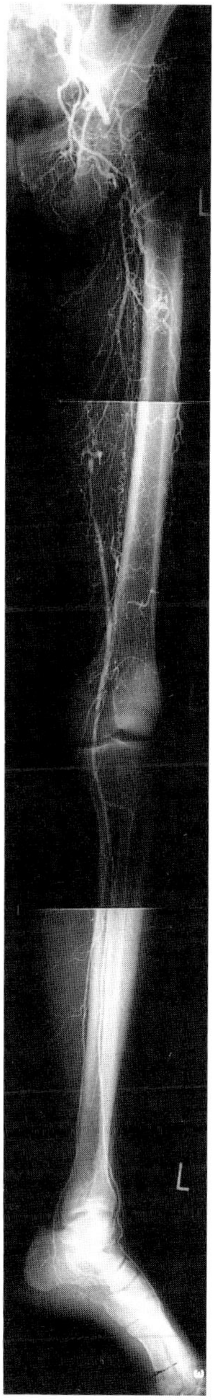

Fig. 10

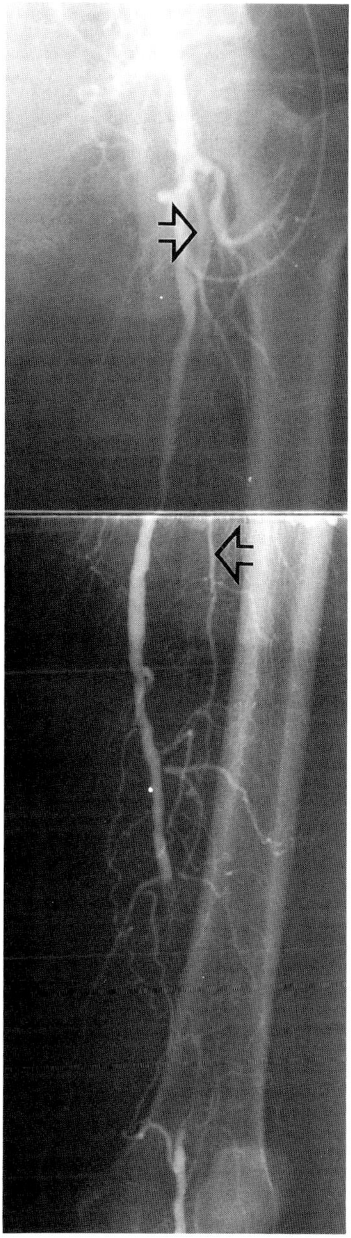

Fig. 11

Fig. 10. Patterns of disease. Proximal deep femoral artery (DFA) stenosis associated with common femoral artery (CFA) occlusion. The distal DFA and thigh collaterals are disease free. The popliteal artery (PA) is reconstituted and there is three-vessel tibial runoff

Fig. 11. Patterns of disease. The main deep femoral artery (DFA) trunk (*arrows*) is diffusely diseased with occlusion of the midsegment

When the preoperative arteriogram is used to predict the likelihood of success following DFA revascularization, the five critical areas to examine are: proximal DFA, distal DFA, DFA (thigh) collaterals, PA, and tibial vessel runoff. When roentgenographically significant proximal DFA disease exists in the presence of a disease-free distal DFA, normal thigh collaterals, a reconstituted popliteal segment, and at least one normal tibial vessel, DFA revascularization will predictably relieve distal ischemia (Fig. 10). Mitchell et al. (1979) have shown that whenever one of those "optimal" arteriographic findings is not present, relief of distal ischemia by isolated profundaplasty is far less likely.

The first arteriographic requisite is hemodynamically significant disease of the proximal DFA. Although some have argued that the undiseased DFA orifice represents a functional stenosis in the presence of concomitant SFA occlusion, essentially all authors now feel that profundaplasty will not be beneficial in the absence of roentgenographically significant atherosclerotic disease of the proximal DFA relative to the distal undiseased artery.

The importance of a normal distal DFA and thigh collaterals has also been emphasized. Fernandes e Fernandes et al. (1978) found a direct correlation between good collateral vessels and success. Andersen et al. (1978) pointed out that successful revascularization required a major descending branch of the DFA reconstituting the genicular branches of the popliteal artery. Stoney (1978) commented that disease in the efferent portion of the DFA collateral vessels proximal to the reconstituted PA was associated with failure. Taylor et al. (1981) also noted that complete absence of collateral vessels around the knee was associated with an unsuccessful result.

Reconstitution of a relatively normal PA is crucial if DFA revascularization is to relieve distal ischemia, and profundaplasty is relatively contraindicated if the PA is occluded or severely diseased. Cotton and Roberts (1975) reported 87% successful relief of distal ischemia by DFA revascularization in patients who were candidates for femoropopliteal bypass, as opposed to 33% success when the PA was occluded or badly diseased. Many others have commented on the importance of patency of the PA, particularly in the absence of iliac disease when profundaplasty alone is being considered.

The quality of the tibial vessels also has a critical influence on the success or failure of DFA revascularization. Morris-Jones and Jones (1974) found a direct relationship between the number of patent tibial vessels and successful relief of ischemia following DFA revascularization. Kalman et al. (1990) and Bernhard et al.

(1976) have also reported that good outflow (two or three patent tibial arteries) was associated with a significantly higher success rate than poor outflow (one or no tibial arteries patent).

Conclusions

Roentgenographic assessment of the DFA requires an understanding of normal anatomy, common anatomical variants, and collateral pathways. When atherosclerosis involves the lower extremity, the DFA is frequently found to be disease free. Furthermore, atherosclerotic involvement of the DFA, when present, is usually restricted to the proximal segment. DFA revascularization, therefore, is frequently possible. Relief of distal ischemia by DFA revascularization, however, will depend on the quality of the outflow tract.

References

Andersen CA, Rich NM, Collins GJ, McDonald PT (1978) Limb salvage by extended profunda femoris revascularization. Am Surg 100: 44–48

Beales JS, Adcock FA, Frawley JS et al (1971) The radiological assessment of disease of the profunda femoris artery. Br J Radiol 44: 854–859

Bernhard VM, Ray LI, Militello JM (1976) The role of angioplasty of the profunda femoris artery in revascularization of the ischemic limb. Surg Gynecol Obstet 142: 840–844

Cotton LT, Roberts VC (1975) Extended deep femoral angioplasty: an alternative to femoropopliteal bypass. Br J Surg 62: 340–343

Fernandes e Fernandes J, Nicolaides AN, Angelides NA, Gordon-Smith IC (1978) An objective assessment of common femoral endarterectomy and profundaplasty in patients with superficial femoral occlusion. Surgery 83: 313–318

Haimovici H (1967) Patterns of arteriosclerotic lesions of the lower extremity. Arch Surg 95: 918–933

Haimovici H, Shapiro JH, Jacobson HG (1960) Serial femoral arteriography in occlusive disease: clinical-roentgenologic considerations with a new classification of occlusive patterns. Am J Roentgenol 83: 1042–1062

Kalman PG, Johnston KW, Walker PM (1990) The current role of isolated profundaplasty. J Cardiovasc Surg 31: 107–111

Margulis AR, Nice CM Jr, Murphy TO (1957) Arteriographic manifestations of peripheral occlusive vascular disease: with the report of two new signs. Am J Roentgenol 78: 273–282

Martin P, Frawley JE, Barabas AP, Rosengarten DS (1972) On the surgery of atherosclerosis of the profunda femoris artery. Surgery 71: 182–189

Mitchell RA, Bone GE, Bridges R, Pamajzl MJ, Fry WJ (1979) Patient selection for isolated profundaplasty: arteriographic correlates of operative results. Am J Surg 138: 912–919

Morris-Jones W, Jones CD (1974) Profundoplasty in the treatment of femoropopliteal occlusion. Am J Surg 127: 680–686

Stoney RJ (1978) Discussion of David TE, Dresher AD: Extended profundaplasty for limb salvage. Surgery 84: 758–763

Taylor LM Jr, Baur GM, Eidemiller LR, Porter JM (1981) Extended profundaplasty. Indications and techniques with results of 46 procedures. Am J Surg 141: 539–542

Thompson BW, Read RC, Campbell GS, Slayden JE, Boyd CM (1976) The role of profundaplasty in revascularization of the lower extremity. Am J Surg 132: 710–715

Towne JB, Rollins DL (1986) Profundaplasty: its role in limb salvage. Surg Clin Am 66: 403–414

6 Indications for Profundaplasty

V.M. BERNHARD

The indications for lower extremity revascularization through the deep femoral artery (DFA) are based on well-established anatomical and physiologic principles. The DFA serves a dual purpose in the economy of lower extremity circulation (Martin and Jamieson 1974; Bernhard et al. 1976). Primarily, it is the main arterial conduit to supply blood to the muscles and other structures of the thigh. Its secondary purpose, as the major collateral for the obstructed superficial femoral artery (SFA), derives from its axial location parallel to the SFA and its length, which can bridge the distance between the common femoral (CFA) and the popliteal vessels. The numerous connections between the distal perforating branches and the genicular vessels establish a rich collateral network to the popliteal artery (PA). When the PA is also occluded, the genicular branches exploit their connections through the recurrent branches of the tibial arteries to reestablish blood flow to the calf. Proximal DFA branches, primarily the medial and lateral circumflex vessels, provide collateral continuity with the pelvis through the cruciate anastomosis to the hypogastric (internal iliac) arteries as well as to the deep epigastric and circumflex iliac vessels in the lower abdominal wall and flank (Martin and Jamieson 1974). These extensive collateral networks leading to and issuing from the DFA establish this artery as the most important alternative for maintaining the vascular integrity of the ischemic lower extremity to compensate for multilevel disease with varying degrees of obstruction in the iliac artery, CFA, SFA, and PA.

The DFA collateral connections to the hypogastric artery have an important role of providing retrograde flow to the pelvic viscera, distal spinal cord, and the buttocks when hypogastric artery perfusion is compromised by arteriosclerosis or surgical obliteration for aneurysmal disease. Failure to recognize the importance of these collaterals and ensure their effective function by profundaplasty may lead to buttock and distal colon necrosis, penile necrosis and paraplegia, or to hip claudication, even though distal limb circulation is adequate (Iliopoulos et al. 1989; Cikrit et al. 1991).

A further important anatomical consideration is the propensity for the DFA and its major branches to undergo progressive dilatation in response to the increased flow as a consequence of decreased peripheral resistance at the arteriolar level imposed by exercise and chronic peripheral ischemia. This widening of the DFA is frequently evident on arteriograms of extremities in which this vessel has been required to serve as the natural bypass for an obstructed SFA.

The fact that these propitious anatomical relationships have physiologic significance has been demonstrated by physiologic studies which clearly show that the flow capacity of the DFA can increase significantly to meet the demands of the calf and foot. Waibel and Wolff (1966) demonstrated a fall in popliteal pressure when the DFA was temporarily clamped in the presence of chronic SFA occlusion. Strandness (1970), Martin and Jamieson (1974), and Bernhard et al. (1976) have demonstrated increased DFA flow by direct operative measurements. The volume of flow through an aortofemoral graft limb with runoff limited to the DFA due to chronic SFA obstruction is equal to the flow which can be measured when the SFA is patent, both before and after vasodilation procedure by the intra-arterial administration of papaverine. Furthermore, flow through the DFA under these circumstances is equal to twice the flow which can usually be measured through a femoral–popliteal bypass. Fernandes e Fernandes et al. (1978) and others (Strandness 1970; David and Drezner 1978; Pearce and Kempczinski 1984) have further demonstrated by noninvasive means that distal perfusion is improved to a significant degree following restoration of flow through the DFA.

Application of these anatomical and physiologic principles to improve extremity circulation depends upon identification of those patients in whom these potentials can be effectively exploited. In order to define indications, it is most convenient to separate patients who require limb revascularization into two categories: those who require an inflow procedure in addition to profundaplasty and those for whom DFA repair is performed as an isolated procedure. The most common application of profundaplasty is in patients with aortoiliac as well as common and SFA obstruction who are undergoing some form of inflow procedure to relieve the more proximal level of obstruction. The second category of patients includes those with limb ischemia due to SFA and PA obstruction in whom aortoiliac inflow is essentially normal. Within this later group are the rare patients who require restoration of DFA continuity following resection of an isolated DFA aneurysm (Markland 1989).

Profundaplasty Combined with Inflow Bypass or Endarterectomy

It is well established that 45%–65% of patients requiring limb revascularization will have combined obstruction involving both the suprainguinal and infrainguinal arteries. When these patients are compared to those with obstruction confined to infrainguinal vessels, the former will generally have less severe atherosclerotic involvement of the popliteal and tibial vessels for a similar degree of calf and pedal ischemia. Given the capacity for hypertrophy and dilatation of the DFA and its rich distal collaterals, this vessel frequently provides a natural bypass to a relatively normal popliteal/tibial bed and therefore can serve as an excellent outflow conduit for any inflow procedure. Under these circumstances, proximal reconstruction by bypass or endarterectomy with restoration of flow through the DFA alone will relieve ischemia to a significant degree in the vast majority of patients. The need for additional bypass to the PA or tibial arteries (Morris et al. 1961; Bernhard et al. 1976; Towne et al. 1981; Brewster et al. 1987) is relatively infrequent and varies between 10% and 30% depending upon the aggressiveness of the reporting surgical group with regard to the perceived need for infrainguinal bypass to relieve claudication. It has been my personal experience (Bernhard 1982) and that of others (Pearce and Kempcinski 1984) that immediate, combined aortofemoral and femoral distal bypass is required in less than 3% of patients with limb-threatening ischemia if adequate inflow revascularization to the DFA has been effectively established. Subsequent bypass may be required to relieve incapacitating claudication or limb-threatening ischemia in 10%–20% of patients who have progressive deterioration of limb circulation due to advancing atherosclerosis.

The purpose of DFA reconstruction as an adjunct to an inflow procedure, therefore, is to ensure unobstructed flow through the DFA to maximize its collateral potential for distal perfusion. The major guiding principle for restoration of DFA flow is to relieve the obstruction, which is usually located at the orifice and/or in the proximal portion of the DFA so that unimpeded central arterial pressure can deliver pulsatile blood flow to the main body of the DFA and its runoff branches.

On occasion, the patient with significant aortoiliac disease will have marginal perfusion through the arterial distribution of the hypogastric and inferior mesenteric vessels. This may place the pelvic organs (Ernst 1985) and distal spinal cord (Picone et al.

1986) in jeopardy in the immediate postoperative period due to inadvertent loss of pelvic collaterals during an aortofemoral bypass. Since it may not be feasible to restore circulation directly to the hypogastric and inferior mesenteric vessels, the pelvic viscera and cord may be dependent to a significant degree upon retrograde flow provided by a profundaplasty to ensure perfusion from the medial and lateral femoral circumflex vessels into the pelvic circulation (Iliopoulos et al. 1989; Cikrit et al. 1991).

The methods for selection of patients who require profundaplasty at the time of an inflow procedure are fairly simple. The arteriogram provides the most important information by indicating the presence of combined inflow and outflow disease and by visualizing the nature, extent, and location of obstructive disease in the proximal portion of the DFA. As noted elsewhere in this monograph (Chap. 5), the oblique angiographic projection is required to place the DFA origin in profile in order to clearly demonstrate its origin, the degree of stenosis, and the extent of disease which is usually located on the posterior wall of the vessel. During the operative procedure, the common femoral arteriotomy should be placed so that the DFA origin can be clearly visualized to demontrate that this vessel is not obstructed by a common femoral plaque extending over or into its orifice or by disease in the proximal vessel which will limit outflow into the distal DFA (Bernhard et al. 1976). The easy passage of a 3.5- to 4-mm probe through the DFA orifice is required to demonstrate that the outflow track is adequately patent. If there is any question of stenosis in the proximal DFA, regardless of its severity, this should be relieved by the most appropriate technique to ensure that aortofemoral limb outflow through the DFA will not be impaired. Recently, duplex scanning of the CFA and DFA has been investigated as a noninvasive preoperative technique to demonstrate the presence and nature of obstruction in these vessels (Marquis et al. 1985; Strauss and Wéber 1990).

An important subgroup in this category of patients with combined aortoiliac and femoral disease are those who have suffered thrombosis of one limb of an aortofemoral, axillofemoral, or femorofemoral graft. In the majority of these patients, it is well established that the cause of graft occlusion is progression of disease at the anastomosis and in the proximal outflow track (Bernhard et al. 1977; Brewster et al. 1987; Agrifoglio et al. 1990). These patients almost invariably have chronic SFA occlusion and have developed fibrointimal hyperplasia or progressing atherosclerosis in the proximal DFA artery. Thrombosis in the early postoperative period is usually due to technical imperfection at the femoral anastomosis or to inadequate outflow in those instances where the femoral anastomosis was originally performed without profundaplasty. Delayed occlusion is generally the result of progression of an unrelieved stenosis or advancing atherosclerosis in the proximal DFA in the months or years following the initial procedure. Restoration of flow through the thrombosed aortofemoral limb can usually be established by balloon catheter thrombectomy; however, this almost always must be complemented by some form of outflow procedure. In the vast majority of patients (70%–95%), this can be accomplished by profundaplasty, which will relieve the obstruction and thus improve flow through the graft (Bernhard et al. 1977; Brewster et al. 1987). The results of surgical restoration of flow by thrombectomy and profundaplasty are excellent, with long-term patency exceeding 75% at 3–5 years.

On occasion, the conventional location for anastomosis at the CFA–DFA junction is difficult to achieve due to severe scarring from previous procedures or the presence of infection in the groin (DePalma et al. 1980; Ouriel et al. 1987). These complicating problems can be avoided by bypassing the groin and performing the distal anastomosis between the aortofemoral graft limb or an alternate route bypass (i.e., axillofemoral, obturator, femorofemoral etc.) to the midportion of the DFA. This segment of the artery is readily approached through an incision in healthy tissue lateral to the sartorius muscle and is a preferred alternative to extending the graft distally to or beyond the knee.

A satisfactory inflow operation, whether an aortofemoral, axillofemoral, or femorofemoral, combined with profundaplasty to ensure unimpaired flow through the DFA will almost invariably relieve the majority of ischemic symptoms in the distal extremity in spite of SFA obstruction (Martin and Jamieson 1974; Goldstone et al. 1978, Towne et al. 1981; Bernhard 1982; Simma et al. 1986; Miksic and Novak 1986). Claudication will be sufficiently relieved to meet the exercise requirements of the majority of patients operated on for this symptom. This is especially true for most elderly patients, whose ambulatory activities will be essentially unimpaired within the spectrum of their normal daily activities. Patients with rest pain will almost invariably be relieved of this symptom, and the majority of superficial ischemic ulcers and some wounds from toe amputations will heal.

Additional bypass to the popliteal or the tibial vessels may be necessary to achieve healing of a persistent deep ischemic ulcer on the ankle or of an extensive debridement or transmetatarsal amputation of the foot. The need for a subsequent infrainguinal bypass will depend upon the quality of the popliteal–tibial runoff tracts distal to the SFA obstruction and the quality of the profundapopliteal collaterals. Since these factors may be difficult to ascertain prior to reestablishing aorto–DFA flow, consideration of a distal bypass should be delayed until the full potential which may be achieved from the revascularized DFA can be assessed after several days or weeks of observation.

Isolated Profundaplasty

The anatomical distribution of disease in patients with obstruction limited to the infrainguinal vessels primarily involves SFA and PA obstruction with a variable degree of involvement of the tibial runoff. In diabetics, atherosclerosis in the vessels below the knee is usually more extensive. Therefore, when the DFA is also obstructed, the potential for collateral compensation is severely compromised (Martin and Jamieson 1974; Bernhard et al. 1976; David and Drezner 1978; Leather et al. 1978; Taylor et al. 1981; Pearce and Kempczinski 1984). Reconstruction of the DFA as an isolated procedure to restore its maximal collateral function under these circumstances may improve distal perfusion sufficiently so that the need for femoral–popliteal or femoral–tibial bypass will not be required (Bernhard et al. 1976; Bernhard 1982). Unfortunately, profundaplasty as an isolated procedure in this situation is much less effective than profundaplasty as a complement to an inflow procedure (Bernhard 1982; Simma et al. 1986; Harward et al. 1988). In the latter, the major obstruction is at the aortoiliac level, which is completely relieved, and the profundaplasty merely ensures adequate runoff into the distal collateral bed. The success of an isolated profundaplasty, however, depends more upon the quality of the runoff through collaterals around the knee and through the tibial vessels into the foot. The potential for significant improvement in pedal perfusion by profundaplasty alone is often severely compromised, since the extent of disease below the knee in patients with similar degrees of pedal ischemia is usually more extensive when the iliac inflow is normal compared to limbs with aortoiliac obstruction combined with SFA disease. It is therefore important to carefully evaluate patients in this category in order to select those in whom isolated profundaplasty will be a more appropriate procedure than bypass to the popliteal or tibial vessels. Several factors must be reviewed, and therefore the decision to perform an isolated profundaplasty rather than femoral–popliteal or femoral–tibial bypass becomes much more complicated.

The distribution and severity of disease in the SFA must be considered initially. Occlusion or stenosis confined to the distal third of this vessel or at the femoral–popliteal junction generally eliminates the DFA as a significant bypass collateral (Sladen and Burgess 1980; Bernhard 1982). Profundaplasty therefore should be considered only in patients who have significant obstructive disease in the proximal SFA.

The degree of stenosis in the DFA should narrow the lumen by at least 50% of its diameter when compared with the apparently nondiseased vessel immediately distal to the point of obstruction (Mitchell et al. 1979; Sladen and Burgess 1980; Bernhard 1982). Theoretical considerations relating to hemodynamic aberrations at the DFA orifice, when only SFA obstruction is present, have been proposed as indications to widen a minimally diseased DFA (Berguer et al. 1975). However, relief of a stenosis of less than 50% in reality produces little improvement in distal perfusion.

Distribution of disease in the DFA should be confined to its orifice or the proximal one third to one half of the vessel where operative repair is feasible (Martin and Jamieson 1974; Bernhard et al. 1976). The distal vessel should be relatively nondiseased with good flow through perforator vessels demonstrated by angiography. Atherosclerosis which involves the middle and distal portion of the DFA, as is frequently the case in diabetics (King et al. 1984), renders this vessel unsuitable for reconstruction.

The quality of the popliteal and/or tibial runoff must be sufficient to permit the improved flow through the DFA to reach the pedal circulation (David and Drezner 1987; Mitchell et al. 1979; Taylor et al. 1981; Bernhard 1982). This is analogous to the quality of outflow required for a femoral–popliteal or femoral–tibial bypass. Ideally, the distal half of the PA should have a relatively unobstructed lumen with at least one fully patent tibial vessel in direct continuity with an intact pedal arch. When this extent of runoff is present, the improved flow introduced into the DFA will encounter increased resistance only at the level of the profunda-popliteal collateral bed. However, when the popliteal-tibial runoff is also impaired, improved DFA flow must traverse at least two high-resistance collateral beds to reach the foot. The extent of improvement in pedal perfusion under these circumstances may not be sufficient to salvage the distal limb in the patient with ischemic ulceration or necrosis. Direct bypass to a patent distal tibial, peroneal, or pedal artery will usually be required when the popliteal and proximal tibial vessels are also occluded.

The quality of the collateral connection between the DFA and the popliteal–tibial runoff is critical for success of an isolated profundaplasty. Arteriography, which demonstrates large connections with rapid flow, may provide sufficient information to indicate that profundaplasty will be effective if the inflow is repaired and the outflow is satisfactory. However, this study depends upon the quality of the arteriogram, the quantity and rate of dye injection, and the timing of the filming sequence. These variables are often difficult, if not impossible, to achieve in a given patient and at best present only a static, unidimensional image.

Noninvasive vascular testing, employing Doppler-derived segmental limb pressure measurements, may provide a more reliable method for determining the adequacy of these collaterals. In 1980, Boren et al. presented the concept of the profundapopliteal collateral index (PPCI) and demonstrated a fairly reliable correlation between this index and the success or failure of isolated profundaplasty. The index is derived by measurement of the systolic pressure above the knee (AKSP) and below the knee (BKSP) and application of the following formula:

$$\frac{\text{AKSP} - \text{BKSP}}{\text{AKSP}} = \text{PPCI}$$

This index merely identifies the severity of the pressure gradient between these two levels. If the index is less than 0.2, the pressure gradient is minimal, suggesting that collaterals are excellent and healing is likely to occur. On the other hand, if the index is 0.5 or greater, the likelihood for healing is zero. This concept has been verified by Ouriel et al. (1987) and by our more recent experience (Rollins et al. 1985).

Other factors which bear upon the indication for isolated profundaplasty include the severity of limb ischemia as determined by symptomatology and physical findings (Bernhard et al. 1976). Repair of a tight DFA stenosis, with good DFA popliteal collaterals, and good to excellent popliteal–tibial runoff is likely to produce significant relief of claudication, although not complete relief of this symptom. Patients with mild to moderate rest pain will also be relieved, although some disability from continued claudication will persist. The presence of severe ischemic ulceration or necrosis is often associated with significant impairment of the popliteal–tibial runoff, and in this group of patients a tibial bypass is more likely to promote healing if the patient has a satisfactory saphenous vein to provide an autogenous conduit and there is a reasonably good distal tibial or peroneal artery in continuity with a pedal arch. Bypass is much more likely to provide direct, high-pressure, pulsatile perfusion to achieve healing in severely ischemic tissues under these circumstances (Harward et al. 1988). However,

Table 1. Choice of operation (occluded superior femoral artery, SFA; normal aortoiliac inflow)

DFA stenosis >50%	Profundapopliteal collateral index <0.5	Popliteal runoff[1]	Procedure recommended
+	+	+	Profundaplasty
+	+	−	Profundaplasty
+	−	+	Femoropopliteal or femorotibial bypass and profundaplasty
+	−	−	Profundaplasty (amputation later?)
−	+/−	+	Femoropopliteal, femorotibial, or sequential bypass
−	+/−	−	Amputation

Adapted from Bernhard (1982), p 260.
DFA, deep femoral artery.
[1] +, good; −, poor.

it is appropriate to perform a profundaplasty in conjunction with a distal bypass if the profundaplasty itself will be of relatively short length and will not unduly prolong the operative procedure. When only a relatively short segment of vein is available, it will be advantageous to perform a proximal profundaplasty and then use the distal DFA as the inflow anastomotic site for bypass to a tibial vessel (Nunez et al. 1988).

When a suitable saphenous or upper extremity venous conduit is not available and a distal bypass must be performed with a prosthetic conduit (i.e., polytetrafluoroetheylene, PTFE), it may by advisable to relieve severe DFA stenosis as the initial procedure and delay bypass with a prosthesis until it has become clear that the DFA repair alone will not be sufficient to salvage the extremity.

Finally, there are patients with no potential for either popliteal, tibial, or pedal bypass for whom profundaplasty is the only method available to improve limb circulation. Although salvage of the ischemic and usually necrotic foot is unlikely in this group, profundaplasty is recommended for these limbs as a preliminary to major amputation. Improved distal perfusion will ensure that an amputation below the knee is most likely to heal, thus improving the potential for ambulation with a prosthesis. In this setting, profundaplasty is performed as an adjunct, preliminary to amputation, to ensure preservation of the knee joint. Without profundaplasty under these circumstances, amputation above the knee will almost certainly be required if DFA flow is impaired, and even at this level, healing may be unreliable (Towne et al. 1981).

The criteria for determining whether isolated profundaplasty should be selected as an alternative to femoral–popliteal or femoral–tibial bypass are presented in Table 1 (Bernhard 1982).

References

Agrifoglio G, Lorenzi G, Castelli PM, Agus GB, Zaretti D, Bavera P (1990) Thrombectomy for late graft limb occlusion: our experience in 182 consecutive cases. J Cardiovasc Surg 31: 617–620

Berguer R, Higgins RF, Cotton LT (1975) Geometry, blood flow, and reconstruction of the deep femoral artery. Am J Surg 130: 68–73

Bernhard VM (1982) Limitations of profunda femoris revascularization. In: Veith FJ (ed) Critical problems in vascular surgery. Appleton-Century-Crofts, New York, pp 251–262

Bernhard VM, Ray LI, Militello JM (1976) The role of angioplasty of the profunda femoris artery in revascularization of the ischemic limb. Surg Gynecol Obstet 142: 840–844

Bernhard VM, Ray LI, Towne JB (1977) The reoperation of choice for aortofemoral graft occlusion. Surgery 82: 867–874

Brewster DC, Meier GH, Darling RC, Moncure AC, LaMuraglia GM, Abbott WM (1987) Reoperation for aortofemoral graft limb occlusion: optimal methods and long term results. J Vasc Surg 5: 363–374

Boren CH, Towne JB, Bernhard VM, Salles-Cunha S (1980) Profundapopliteal collateral index. A guide to successful profundaplasty. Arch Surg 115: 1366–1372

Cikrit DF, O'Donnell DM, Dalsing MC, Sawchuck AP, Lalka SG (1991) Clinical implications of combined hypogastric and profunda femoral artery occlusion. Am J Surg 162: 137–141

David TE, Drezner AD (1978) Extended profundoplasty for limb salvage. Surgery 84: 758–763

DePalma RG, Malgieri JJ, Rhodes RS, Clowes AW (1980) Profunda femoris bypass for secondary revascularization. Surg Gynecol Obstet 151: 387–390

Ernst CB (1985) Intestinal ischemia following abdominal aortic reconstruction. In: Bernhard VM, Towne JB (eds) Complications in vascular surgery. Grune and Stratton, New York, pp 325–350

Fernandes e Fernandes JF, Nicolaides AN, Angelides NA, Gordon-Smith IC (1978) An objective assessment of common femoral endarterectomy and profundaplasty in patients with superficial femoral occlusion. Surgery 83: 313–318

Goldstone J, Malone JM, Moore WS (1978) Importance of the profunda femoris artery in primary and secondary arterial operations for lower extremity ischemia. Am J Surg 136: 215–220

Harward TR, Bergan JJ, Yao JS, Flinn WR, McCarthy WJ (1988) The demise of primary profundaplasty. Am J Surg 156: 126–129

Iliopoulos JI, Hermreck AS, Thomas JH, Pierce GE (1989) Hemodynamics of the hypogastric arterial circulation. J Vasc Surg 9: 637–642

King TA, DePalma RG, Rhodes RS (1984) Diabetes mellitus and atherosclerotic involvement of the produnda femoris artery. Surg Gynecol Obstet 159: 553–556

Leather RP, Shah DM, Karmody AM (1978) The use of extended profundaplasty in limb salvage. Am J Surg 136: 359–362

Markland CG (1989) Primary atherosclerotic aneurysm of the profunda femoris artery associated with distal embolization. Ann Vasc Surg 3: 389–391

Marquis C, Meister JJ, Meuli R, Mooser E, Mosimann R (1985) Quantitative Messung der Blutströmung mit einem 128-kanaligen Doppler-Gerät. Ultraschall Med 6: 83–89

Martin P, Jamieson C (1974) The rationale for and measurement after profundaplasty. Surg Clin North Am 54: 95–109

Miksic K, Novak D (1986) Profunda femoris revascularization in limb salvage. J Cardiovasc Surg 27: 544–562

Mitchell RA, Bone GE, Bridges R, Pamajz MJ, Fry WJ (1979) Patient selection for isolated profundaplasty. Arteriographic correlates of operative results. Am J Surg 138: 912–919

Morris GC, Edwards E, Cooley DA et al (1961) Surgical importance of profunda femoris artery. Analysis of 102 cases with combined aortoiliac and femoropopliteal exclusive disease treated by revascularization of deep femoral artery. Arch Surg 82: 32–37

Nunez AA, Veith FJ, Collier P, Ascer E, Flores SW, Gupta SK (1988) Direct approaches to the distal portions of the deep femoral artery for limb salvage bypasses. J Vasc Surg 8: 576–581

Ouriel K, DeWeese JA, Ricotta JJ, Green RM (1987) Revascularization of the distal profunda femoris artery in the reconstructive treatment of aortoiliac occlusive disease. J Vasc Surg 6: 217–220

Pearce WH, Kempczinski RF (1984) Extended autogenous profundaplasty and aortofemoral grafting: an alternative to synchronous distal bypass. J Vasc Surg 1: 455–458

Picone AL, Green RM, Ricotta JR, May AG, DeWeese JA (1986) Spinal cord ischemia following operations on the abdominal aorta. J Vasc Surg 3: 94–103

Rollins DL, Towne JB, Bernhard VM et al (1985) Endarterectomized superficial femoral artery as an arterial patch. Arch Surg 120: 267–269

Simma W, Bassiouny H, Hartl P, Brucke P (1986) Evaluation of profundaplasty in reconstructions of combined aortoiliac and femoro-popliteal occlusive disease. J Cardiovasc Surg 27: 141–145

Sladen JG, Burgess JJ (1980) Profundaplasty: expectations and ominous signs. Am J Surg 140: 242–245

Strandness DE (1970) Functional results after revascularization of the profunda femoris artery. Am J Surg 119: 240–245

Strauss AL, Wéber G (1990) Non-invasive determination of the hemodynamic significance vasoconstriction: study of the arteria femoris profunda using ultrasound. Orv Hetil 131: 859–862

Taylor LM, Baur GM, Eidemiller LR, Porter JM (1981) Extended profundaplasty. Indications and techniques with results of 46 procedures. Am J Surg 141: 539–542

Towne JB, Bernhard VM, Rollins DL, Baum PI (1981) Profundaplasty in perspective: limitations in the long-term management of limb ischemia. Surgery 90: 1037–1046

Waibel PP, Wolff G (1966) The collateral circulation in occlusions of the femoral artery; an experimental study. Surgery 60: 912–918

7 Surgical Approaches

M.Y. SUTER

Since Oudot and Cormier's first description of the possibility of distal revascularization of the lower limb through the deep femoral artery (DFA) in 1953 (Oudot and Cormier 1953), the importance of this vessel in vascular reconstruction procedures has risen constantly. In 1957, Henry described the surgical approach to the proximal DFA (Henry 1957). This approach was merely the distal extension of the incision used to expose the femoral bifurcation. Hershey and Auer (1974) gave a precise description of an extended surgical approach which permits exposure of the DFA as far its distal branches. This approach is now the standard one for most procedures on the DFA. Modifications of it have been described, including an incision which exposes only the middle and distal thirds of the DFA. A posterior approach, as well as a medial approach, have been described, which can be used in circumstances that will be discussed below.

This chapter will first describe the standard approach to the whole trunk of the DFA. The other modalities to expose the DFA will then be discussed, with special emphasis on their indications and limitations.

Exposure of the Whole Trunk of the Deep Femoral Artery

The anteromedial approach to the whole trunk of the DFA as first described by Hershey and Auer (1974) is now the standard one for most procedures of DFA reconstruction or profundaplasty. The DFA can be readily exposed from its origin at the bifurcation of the common femoral artery (CFA) down to its distal branches. As in most cases the distal limit of endarterectomy and profundaplasty or the exact site of anastomosis cannot been determined preoperatively; the use of an incision, which can be extended as far distally as needed, is often helpful for most procedures.

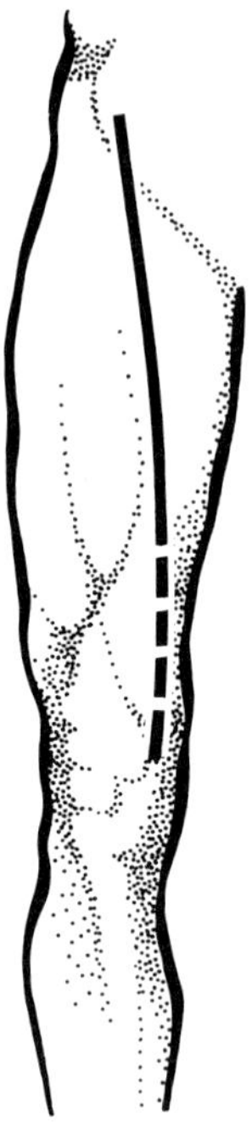

Fig. 1. Line of skin incision for the exposure of the whole trunk of the deep femoral artery (DFA)

The patient is placed in the supine position. The extent of the surgical field and draping should permit free intraoperative hip and knee flexion with external rotation of the thigh. A slight elevation of the contralateral hip may be helpful. The so-called frog position permits relaxation and retraction of the anterior muscles of the thigh, improving the visibility of the deeply located DFA.

The skin incision is on a theoretical line which begins two fingerbreadths medial to the anterior superior iliac spine and extends distally to the medial border of the patella (Fig. 1). Dissection of the femoral bifurcation is first undertaken. The deep fascia is incised and the medial border of the sartorius muscle is identified and separated from the adipose tissue in the groin. The sartorius muscle is retracted laterally and the fat medially (Fig. 2). In this way, the lymph nodes in the groin are not entered and the risk of postoperative lymphorrhea is reduced. The vascular sheath is then opened and the CFA is dissected free from the inguinal ligament down to its bifurcation. Care must be taken not to damage the side branches, which can play a major role in the collateral circulation, and especially the lateral femoral circumflex artery. This vessel can arise from the lateral aspect of the CFA in 5%–15% of cases (Schwilden and van Dongen 1987). The medial femoral circumflex artery can originate from the CFA in 30%–

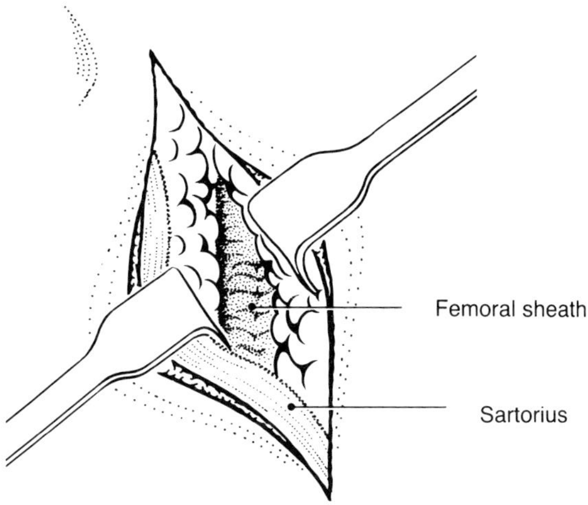

Fig. 2. Exposure of the whole trunk of the deep femoral artery (DFA). Approach to the common femoral artery (CFA), the sartorius muscle being retracted laterally

40% of cases, usually on its posterior aspect (Schwilden and van Dongen 1987).

The bifurcation of the CFA is usually located 3–5 cm below the inguinal ligament. A discrete narrowing of the diameter of the trunk can indicate the beginning of the superficial femoral artery (SFA). The origin of the DFA is usually on the posterior or lateral aspect of the CFA. It is easy to recognize as a gentle traction is applied medially and anteriorly on two loops placed around the CFA and the SFA (Fig. 3). The deep fascia is divided and the dissection of the DFA begins. The first 2 cm run posteriorly and laterally. At this level, one or two venae comitantes and the lateral femoral circumflex vein cross over the DFA. They are ligated and divided. In rare instances (approximately 3%), they run posterior to the DFA; if damaged, they cause troublesome bleeding. The origin of the medial and lateral circumflex arteries are usually found on this portion of the DFA. Their dissection must be carried out carefully and small arterial loops passed around them.

As the dissection progresses distally, the rectus femoris and sartorius muscle are retracted laterally. After the first 2 cm, the DFA curves medially and then runs distally, slightly posterior and lateral to the SFA on the anterior surface of the pectineus and adductor muscles. The deep femoral vein lies in front of the DFA up to its junction with the superficial femoral vein. When the superficial femoral venous system is not obstructed, the deep femoral vein can be ligated and divided to facilitate exposure. At

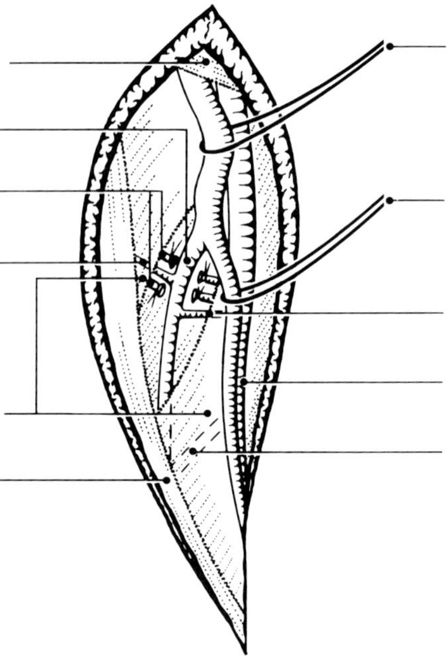

Fig. 3. Exposure of the whole trunk of the deep femoral artery (*DFA*). Dissection of the origin of the DFA. *CFA*, common femoral artery; *SFA*, superficial femoral artery

this point, the motor nerves to the sartorius and rectus femoris muscles are identified and reclined together with their muscles. The motor nerve to the vastus medialis muscle runs lateral to the DFA along the first 10 cm. More distally, it lies closer to the artery, but still can be retracted laterally.

Six to eight centimeters below the origin of the DFA, the first perforating artery, and a few centimeters more distally, the second one are easily identified. About 12–15 cm from its beginning, the DFA passes behind the adductor longus muscle. This muscle can be partially or even completely divided vertically to allow further exposure. The third perforating artery is isolated at this level. The most distal portion of the DFA (fourth perforating artery) is close to the linea aspera of the femur, posterior to the adductor magnus muscle, and not accessible through this anteromedial approach (Fig. 4).

The DFA should only be dissected as far as necessary and the perforating arteries, as well as its other small muscular branches, should be spared carefully. In this way, the collateral circulation to the distal part of the limb will remain intact. Dissection of 3 cm is enough to perform an anastomosis between two small clamps.

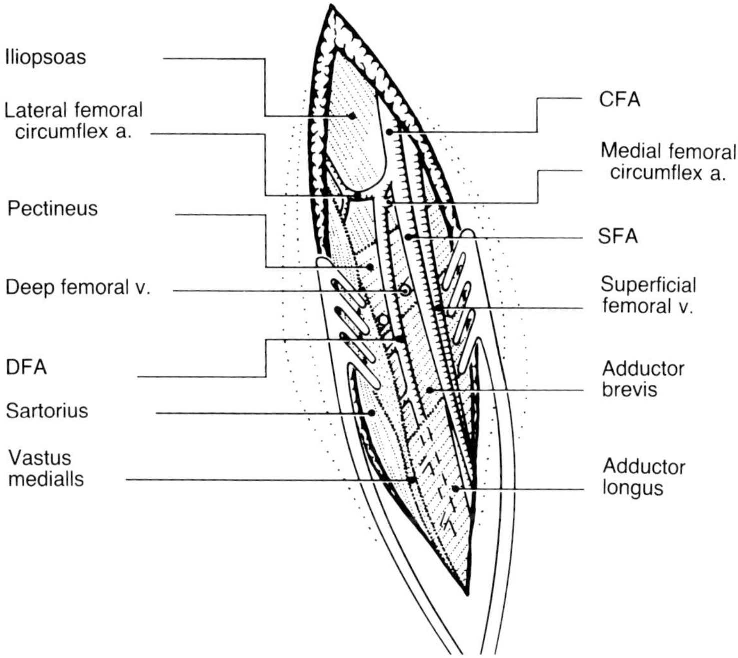

Fig. 4. Complete exposure of the whole trunk of the deep femoral artery (*DFA*). The adductor longus muscle has not been divided. *CFA*, common femoral artery; *SFA*, superficial femoral artery

Meticulous closure of the wound is especially important in the groin. A suction drain is placed between the muscles, but not in contact with the artery, and the aponeurosis is closed loosely with interrupted sutures. The subcutanous tissue is then approximated in the same way, usually with a second suction drain. Closure of the skin must be meticulous, with interrupted sutures. The stitches must be loose enough to prevent ischemia. For the same reason, continuous running sutures should be avoided.

Anterior Approach to the Middle and Distal Thirds of the Deep Femoral Artery

If local conditions in the groin (infection, dense scarring following former procedures or radiotherapy) preclude the dissection of the femoral bifurcation and the proximal DFA and thus profundaplasty, direct exposure of the medial and distal thirds of the DFA is possible through a more distal incision that avoids the groin. The

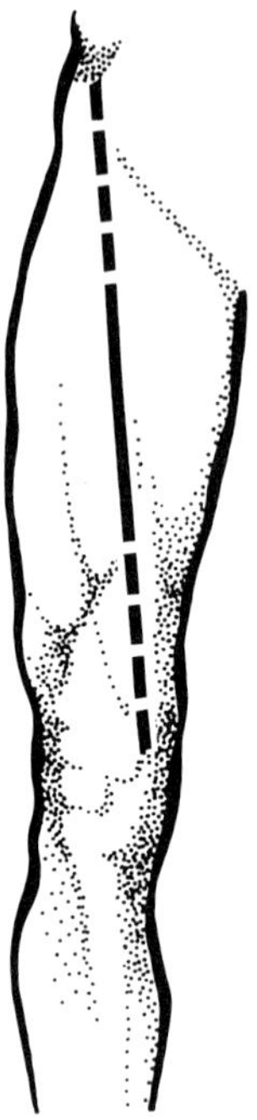

Fig. 5. Line of skin incision for the anterior approach to the medial and distal deep femoral artery (DFA)

DFA can thus be used as the recipient or the origin of bypass grafts. To expose the DFA at this level, one possible way is to use the distal portion of the approach described above for the whole trunk, in which the sartorius and rectus femoris muscles are rectracted laterally (Hershey and Auer 1974). An alternative method was described in 1970 by Bouchet (1970, 1976) and later by Gillot et al. (1975): the skin is incised slightly more anteriorly on the thigh, and the sartorius muscle is reclined medially (Cormier).

The patient is placed in the supine position. The draping must permit intraoperative flexion of the hip and knee and external rotation of the thigh. The skin is incised along the line that joins the anterior superior iliac spine and the medial border of the patella. The incision begins about 12 cm below the iliac spine and extends approximately 12 cm distally to the midthigh (Fig. 5). It must be located over the rectus femoris muscle and not over the groove between the vastus medialis and the sartorius muscles. The deep fascia is divided and the rectus femoris muscle exposed (Fig. 6). The dissection proceeds along the medial border of this muscle and, deeper, along the medial border of the vastus medialis muscle. The sartorius muscle is retracted medially. The SFA is very close to the DFA in the midthigh and therefore, to avoid confusion, care

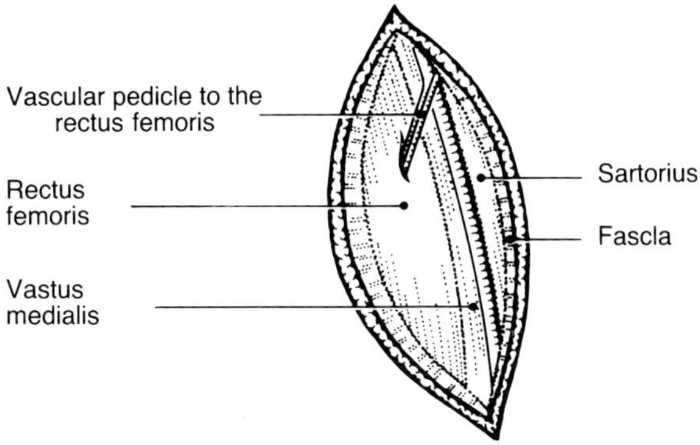

Fig. 6. Anterior approach to the medial and distal deep femoral artery (DFA). The superficial fascia has been divided

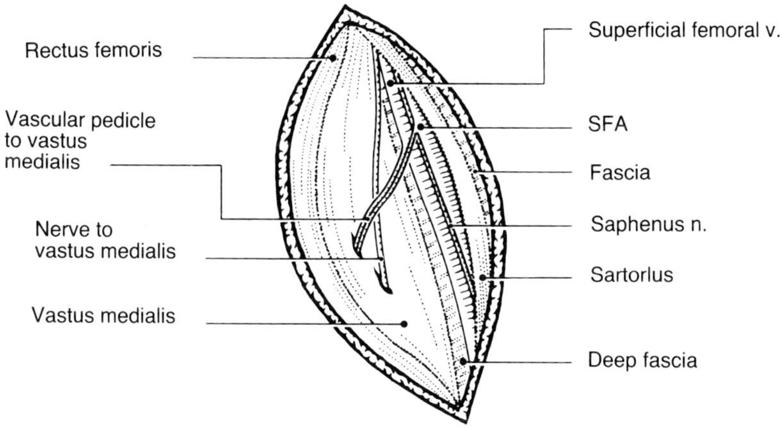

Fig. 7. Anterior approach to the medial and distal deep femoral artery (DFA). Dissection between the sartorius and the vastus medialis muscles. The vascular pedicle and the nerve to this muscle can be seen. *SFA*, superficial femoral artery

must be taken to keep close to the vastus medialis muscle. Its nerve must be identified and reclined laterally with the muscle. As the dissection is deepened (Fig. 7), the vascular pedicle to the vastus medialis muscle is seen, originating from the superficial femoral vessels. This pedicle can be ligated and divided. At this point of the dissection, a self-retaining retractor becomes very helpful. The DFA is identified in the groove between the vastus medialis and the adductor brevis muscles, usually at the level of the second perforating artery (Fig. 8). The arterial trunk is accompanied by one or two deep femoral veins, which can be spared in

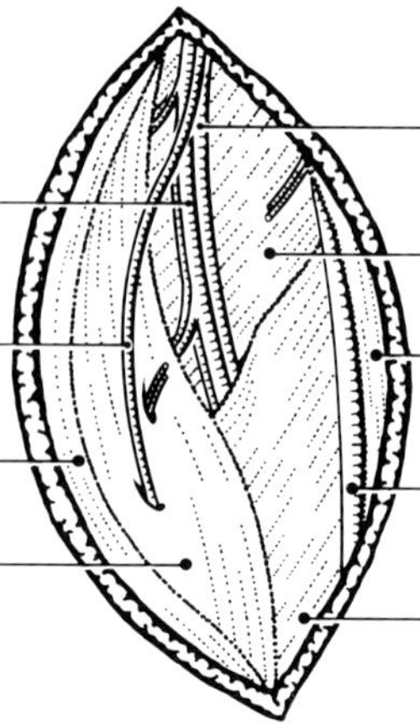

Fig. 8. Anterior approach to the medial and distal deep femoral artery (*DFA*). The artery is prepared between the muscles. The motor nerve to the vastus medialis is carefully preserved. *SFA*, superficial femoral artery

most instances. On the other hand, the venae comitantes that cross the DFA must be ligated and divided. A sufficient portion of the DFA is easily dissected free at this level to permit the performance of an anastomosis. If necessary, the fibers of the adductor longus muscle are divided vertically to provide further exposure. Proximally, exposure is usually sufficient and dissection does not need to extend as far as the first perforating artery. At this level, the DFA is usually of sufficient caliber to permit a good anastomosis.

Closure of the wound is done as described above.

Medial Approach to the Distal Deep Femoral Artery

When the distal portion of the DFA is used as the origin of a bypass to a more distal vessel, it can be exposed through a medial incision as is used to remove the saphenous vein (Buxton et al. 1978).

The patient is placed in the supine position. Draping must permit flexion and external rotation of the hip. The skin is incised medially, along the course of the saphenous vein, which is prepared and removed, unless an in situ bypass is foreseen. The deep fascia is then divided and the sartorius muscle is retracted anterolaterally. The dissection is deepened between the adductor longus and the adductor magnus muscles. In the distal portion of the incision, the SFA is first seen in front of the adductor longus muscle and then passing behind the adductor magnus through the adductor's hiatus. The distal DFA lies anterior to the adductor brevis and adductor magnus muscles, but posterior to the adductor longus muscle. It is located close to the femur, from which it is separated by the insertion of the vastus medialis muscle.

Closure of the wound is performed as described above.

Posterior Approach to the Distal Deep Femoral Artery

Sometimes, extended fibrosis or infection in the groin and anterior thigh preclude the dissection of the femoral bifurcation and the proximal DFA. Therefore, their use for procedures such as profundaplasty or bypass is not possible. Fibrosis in the groin can make dissection of the femoral bifurcation very difficult. Even if the proximal anastomosis of a bypass is performed on the common or external iliac artery, extended fibrosis around the bypass can jeopardize its long-term permeability. If there is infection in the groin, an extra-anatomic bypass is mandatory for distal revascularization procedures in case of obstruction of the SFA. Its origin is usually the axillary artery. The long-term permeability of such a long unilateral extra-anatomic bypass is poor, which usually makes its use as a temporary limb-salvage procedure time limited.

If the SFA is obstructed and the permeability of the iliac arteries, the CFA, and the DFA is good, the distal portion of the DFA can be used as the origin of a bypass. Exposure of this distal part of the DFA is possible through a posterior approach on the thigh (Farley et al. 1964). It must be emphasized that the DFA must be of good quality and caliber down to its distal third, because more proximal exposure of the DFA is not possible with this posterior approach. These limited possibilities make its use of value only in limb-salvage surgery, if there is no other choice. Another possible indication is the availability of only a short venous segment to bypass the knee.

With the patient in the prone position, the knee is slightly flexed to provide relaxation of the posterior muscles of the thigh. The skin is incised vertically over the groove between the semitendinosus and biceps muscles. The fascia is divided and the two muscles are separated by blunt dissection. The long head of the biceps is rectracted laterally, and the sciatic nerve is seen. This nerve is also reclined laterally. The semitendinosus, together with the underlying semimembranosus, is retracted medially.

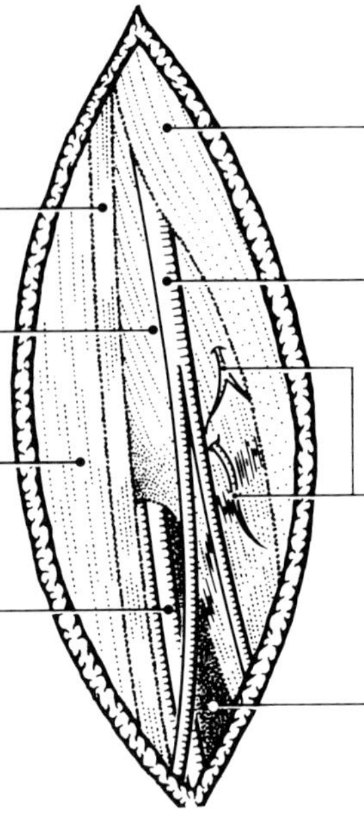

Fig. 9. Posterior approach to the distal deep femoral artery (*DFA*)

A large muscular branch of the DFA will be found, coming through the adductor magnus muscle (Fig. 9). This vessel is dissected proximally toward the DFA, which is located on the other side of the adductor magnus muscle. The fibers of this muscle must be split or divided to provide good exposure. The distal portion of the DFA can then be freed from the intermuscular septum, close to the linea aspera of the femur. Its diameter usually permits a good anastomosis to be performed. The wound is closed according to the principles that have already been described.

References

Bouchet A (1970) Les pontages veineux fémoro-poplités implantés en haut sur la portion moyenne de l'artère fémorale profonde. Lyon Chir 66: 451–454

Bouchet A (1976) A propos de la voie d'abord de l'artère fémorale profonde distale. J Chir 111: 553–560

Buxton B, Reeves L, Roberts AK (1978) Distal profunda femoris to popliteal artery bypass for patients with a short length of long saphenous vein. Surgery 83: 245–247

Cormier JM. Chirurgie du carrefour fémoral et de l'artère fémorale profonde. In: Encyclopédie médico-chirurgicale, techniques chirurgicales. Chirurgie vasculaire. Editions Techniques, Paris, 43070, 4.8.12

Farley HH, Kiser JC, Hitchcock CR (1964) Profunda femoris-popliteal shunt. Ann Surg 160: 23–25

Gillot C, Frileux C, Pillot-Bienaymel (1975) Abord direct pour pontage de l'artère fémorale profonde distale. La voie sus-médiocrurale. J Chir 110: 45–60

Henry AK (1957) Extensile exposure. Livingstone, Edinburgh, pp 227–241

Hershey FB, Auer AI (1974) Extended surgical approach to the profunda femoris artery. Surg Gynecol Obstet 138: 88–90

Oudot J, Cormier JM (1953) La localisation la plus fréquente de l'artérite segmentaire: celle de la femorale superficielle. Presse Med 61: 1361–1364

Schwilden EA, van Dongen RJAM (1987) Engriffe an der arteria profunda femoris. In: Heberer G, van Dongen RJAM (eds) Gefässchirurgie. Springer, Berlin Heidelberg New York, pp 457–473

8 Deep Femoral Artery Revascularization

M.P. Merlini

Following the description of the surgical approach of the deep femoral artery (DFA), this chapter and the subsequent ones are devoted to the surgical techniques and their specific indications. The current chapter deals with revascularization of the DFA. In this term, one must include all the techniques which improve blood flow at the ostium of this artery (Schwilden and van Dongen 1987; Fig. 1). They are not techniques concerning the DFA itself: the trunk of this artery and even the ostium are not affected. Revascularization improves proximal flow. One must therefore differentiate between revascularization and profundaplasty (Chap. 9).

Profundaplasty improves DFA flow by enlarging it from the ostium over a variable length and can be limited (above the first perforating artery) or extensive (beyond the first perforating artery; Iliopoulos et al. 1985; Rollins et al. 1985). Revascularization is also differentiated from reconstruction (Chap. 10). Reconstruction aims at improving DFA blood flow using a technique other than plasty. This generally means a bypass from the common femoral artery (CFA) to the distal DFA. The terms "revascularization" and "profundaplasty" are applied in the literature in accordance with the definition given in this book (Paes and Hamann 1989; Edwards et al. 1989, McCoy et al. 1989; Towne and Rollins 1986). The term "reconstruction" is used in the literature with less precision than in this text (Feldhaus et al. 1985; Miksic and Novak 1986). The term "distal revascularization" is also occasionally found in the literature (Nunez et al. 1988; Ouriel et al. 1987; Jausseran et al. 1991) and applies to proximal bypasses, the distal anastomosis of which is onto the DFA below the first perforating artery. This term is appropriate, but it is not a revascularization in the strict sense applied in this book (increase inflow at the takeoff of the DFA). For this reason, distal revascularization is considered in the chapter on reconstruction (Chap. 10). The above-mentioned definitions are repeated at the beginning of Chap. 9.

The DFA is the main collateral vessel in the thigh. Through its main trunk, the network of interperforating arches, and the de-

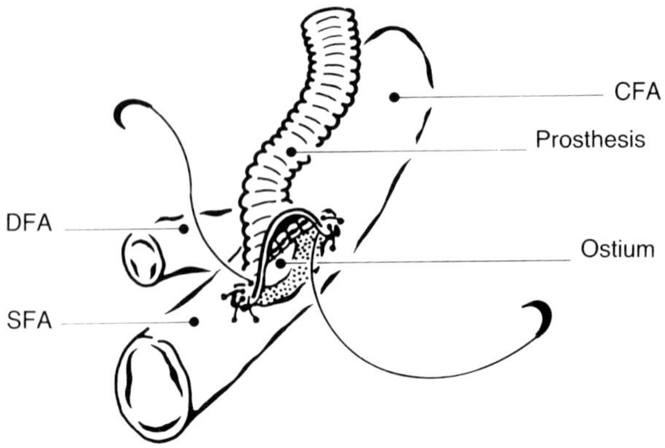

Fig. 1. Deep femoral artery (*DFA*) revascularization: blood flow is improved at the ostium. *CFA*, common femoral artery; *SFA*, superficial femoral artery

scending branch of the lateral femoral circumflex artery, it can completely compensate for a superficial femoral artery (SFA) obstruction (Bernhard et al. 1976). The DFA is also a natural suitable route in the event of proximal obstruction (aortoiliac). In this case, the collateral parietal and visceral system develops and uses the course of this artery to vascularize the lower limb (Chap. 3; Krahl et al. 1954; Friedenberg and Perez 1965; Iliopoulos et al. 1989; Iliopoulos et al. 1990; Krupski et al. 1984; Dietzek et al. 1990; Gaylis 1992).

If, in the thigh, obstruction of the SFA can be compensated by the DFA, aortoiliac occlusion is rarely completely compensated for via the lumbopelvic collateral system and is, in the majority of cases, symptomatic. The possibility of achieving adequate revascularization of the lower limb by the DFA in the event of an aortoiliac obstruction explains the interest in revascularization techniques.

Indication for Deep Femoral Artery Revascularization

The clinical examination of the patient by palpation of the femoral pulses and auscultation of murmurs is subjective in the assessment of aortoiliac stenoses. The qualitative sensation of the pulse depends upon the patient's systolic pressure, artery elasticity, and the thickness of the inguinal subcutaneous tissue. Asymmetry of the femoral pulses or very weak pulsation is the clinical sign of advanced proximal stenosis (Kitslaar et al. 1988). Palpation alone cannot, however, determine a critical stenosis requiring revascularization.

Segmental arterial plethysmography measures the increase in limb volume with the cardiac cycle. Analysis of the aortoiliac segment, however, comes up against technical difficulties as the cuff of the plethysmograph covers the first segment of the SFA no matter how highly placed it may be on the thigh. Thus, the curve analyzes not only the aortoiliac segment, but often its summation with the SFA. As a matter of fact, obstruction of the SFA results in a dampening of the pulse volume recording (PVR). In certain centers, equipment has been developed which enables isolated pneumatic compression of the CFA (Barringer et al. 1983) and so avoids these estimation errors. These techniques have a 97% accuracy in aortoiliac stenosis exceeding 50%. However, they are not in widespread use. Arterial plethysmography cannot be used alone as an indication for revascularization.

Investigation by Doppler gives a great deal of information on aortoiliac involvement. Waveform analysis registered at the level of the CFA can be related to a hemodynamically significant stenosis of this segment: disappearance of the negative phase (absence of reverse diastolic flow) can be correlated in 96% of cases with a stenosis exceeding 50% (Persson et al. 1981).

The pulsatility index (PI) quantatively analyzes the Doppler wave. The PI is the ratio of the peak-to-peak frequency difference to the mean frequency during the cardiac cycle. It is automatically calculated with current equipment. At the level of the CFA, the PI is between 5 and 10. These values fall in stenoses and suggest inflow disease with a specificity and a sensitivity of 75%–95%, respectively (Bagi et al. 1990; Johnston 1987). PI is, however, influenced by distal stenoses and falsely low values are obtained for the CFA. Thus, Doppler waveform analysis cannot be used alone in assessment of the aortoiliac segment for DFA revascularization.

Duplex scanning applied to the aortoiliac segment determines stenoses of more than 50% by doubling the peak systolic velocity and loss of the negative component and by spectral enlargement (Baker 1990). The duplex is as effective as biplanar or digitalized angiography (Legemate et al. 1991) in the detection of stenoses requiring treatment by angioplasty (van der Heijden et al. 1993) or surgery and results in a sensitivity of 82% and a specificity of 92% (Kohler et al. 1987). In certain cases, the duplex even gives a hemodynamic evaluation of the aortoiliac segment similar to the invasive pressure measurement (Sawchuk et al. 1990), i.e., an accuracy of 92%–100%.

Currently, therefore, noninvasive techniques exist for precise analysis of the aortoiliac segment. However, the duplex requires considerable experience and is time consuming. It does not as yet supplant preoperative arteriography, which retains incontestable advantages for the surgeon (see below). The duplex allows, on the other hand, an excellent postoperative follow-up study (Chap. 11; Legemate et al. 1989).

Invasive Investigation of the Aortoiliac Segment

Arteriography is essential for indicating DFA revascularization. Current hemodynamic methods compared to arteriography (Legemate et al. 1991; Bagi et al. 1988; Carpenter et al. 1992; Cossman et al. 1989) have enabled the role of this investigation, its advantages, and its limitations to be reevaluated. Arteriography reveals in a few images the entire vascular tree, the general topography of stenoses and obstructions, and their length. It compares both sides and outlines the lumboiliac, hypogastric, visceral, deep femoral, and genicular collateral networks. Their condition can be appreciated before DFA revascularization. Arteriography is also a method still benefitting from ongoing development (Bettmann 1992). It shows up multilevel stenoses, the hemodynamic burden of which is more severe than that of tight isolated stenoses (Sumner 1989). It is therefore necessary in assessment of multilevel disease. Its limitations are nowadays known: arteriography does not provide hemodynamic information. Single-plane investigation underestimates aortoiliac stenoses. Moreover, biplanar- or oblique-view examination necessitates a supplementary injection of contrast medium, which is potentially harmful in the case of renal insufficiency.

Invasive arterial blood pressure measurement during arteriography or preoperatively is the most objective hemodynamic criterion of aortoiliac stenosis and should be considered as the "gold standard" in DFA revascularization. The finding of a 15% pressure gradient compared with radial blood pressure indicates this revascularization (Flanigan et al. 1984). This assessment can be perfected by intra-arterial injection of 30–50 mg papaverine. Vasodilation due to papaverine refines the diagnosis of aortoiliac lesions and reveals subcritical stenoses. A subcritical stenosis is distinguished by the absence of a pressure gradient at rest and the appearance of a gradient after injection of papaverine. In this event, a central revascularization is also indicated. However, sometimes, in spite of a negative papaverine test, a brachiofemoral gradient appears after femorofemoral or femoropopliteal bypass surgery. This phenomenon occurs in 18% of femorofemoral bypasses and in 8% of femoropopliteal bypasses (Gupta et al. 1990) and is attributed to the opening up of the peripheral vascular bed after the creation of the bypass.

Aortobifemoral Bypass (Fig. 2)

Aortobifemoral bypass has become a technical standard in vascular surgery (Szilagyi et al. 1986). In obstructive disease, the indication might be a disabling claudication or the threat of necrosis. The prostheses used for this type of surgery are manufactured in polyethylene terephtalate (Dacron), a material already in existence for many years. These prostheses have been perfected in both design and manufacture (Guidoin et al. 1992). They have, for example, a concertina-like appearance, enabling their length to be altered during implantation to prevent flattening when they form a slight curve. They are impregnated with collagen, albumin, or gelatin, thus avoiding precoagulation with recipient blood and transparietal hemorrhage after insertion. Experience is also growing in the use

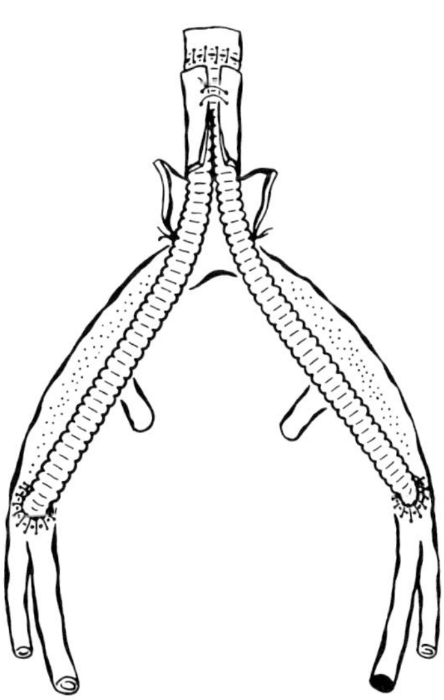

Fig. 2. Aortobifemoral bypass: the proximal anastomosis is performed in an end-to-end fashion; the vertical limb is short with prosthetic bifurcation above native aortoiliac bifurcation

of wide-diameter polytetrafluroethylene (PTFE) prostheses, which are very stable. These do not dilate over the long term.

The surgical approach of choice is a median xiphopubic laparotomy. The proximal anastomosis can be performed end-to-end or end-to-side (Mellière et al. 1990). The former has the advantage of not creating a kink between the aorta and the prosthesis and of diminishing anastomotic turbulence. The posterior peritoneal closure is also easier and reduces the risk of an aortoenteral fistula (Johnston 1990). This anastomosis, however, interrupts native anterograde iliac flow. In this event, iliac flow is provided by the retrograde collateral route from the DFA and the external iliac artery (EIA) (Iliopoulos et al. 1989).

The trunk of the aortobifemoral prosthesis must be cut short, so that the limbs remain as straight as possible. The bifurcation of the prosthesis must occur a few centimeters above the native aortoiliac bifurcation. The proximal anastomosis is achieved using a nonresorbable 2–0 or 3–0 monofilament suture.

The distal anastomosis is performed end-to-side on the distal CFA. Revascularization in the strict sense of the word does not involve any enlargement of the ostium of the DFA. If this is stenosed, femoral arteriotomy can be extended beyond the ostium and the distal anastomosis put onto the distal CFA and the first segment of the DFA. It is therefore a "profundaplasty–revascularization."

The patency of aortobifemoral bypasses is 85%–90% at 5 years and 70%–75% at 10 years (Goldstone 1990). When the SFA is occluded, patency is lower, of the order of 72% at 5 years.

Iliofemoral Bypass (Fig. 3)

In the case of unilateral obstructive disease preferentially involving the EIA, an aortofemoral bypass (Kram et al. 1991) or a unilateral iliofemoral bypass can be considered. Unilateral bypass is, however, controversial. Piotrowski et al. (1988) demonstated the superiority of bilateral bypass both when the SFA is patent as well as when it is occluded. The primary patency at 5 years after aortobifemoral and -unifemoral bypass with a patent SFA is 89% and 36%, respectively. With an occluded SFA it is 72% and 56%. Lorentzen et al. (1990), on the other hand, found that out of 129 unilateral iliofemoral bypass patients followed up for 3 years, only five (3.8%) required subsequent iliac reconstruction of the other

Fig. 3. Iliofemoral bypass: end-to-side prosthesis implanted to cross an external iliac artery (EIA) obstruction

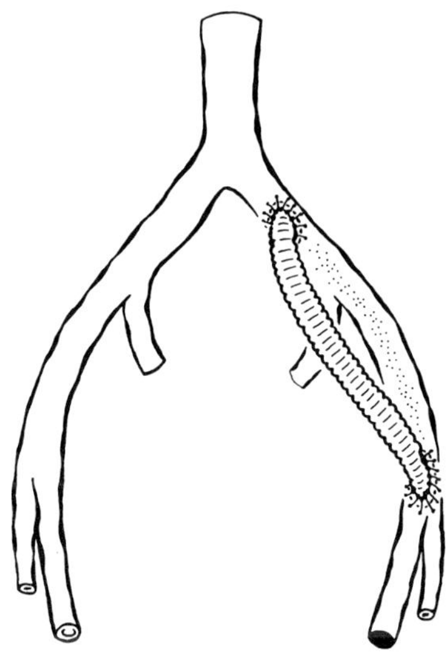

side. Furthermore, the development of transluminal angioplasty now limits the indications for unilateral bypass.

The surgical approach is the retroperitoneal route for the iliac artery and a vertical inguinal incision for the femoral artery. The material used can be a PTFE (8 mm in diameter) or polyethylene terephtalate. The proximal anastomosis is carried out in the end-to-side position with 4–0 monofilament suture. The distal anastomosis is carried out on the CFA with an extension of profundaplasty if the ostium of the DFA diseased.

Kalman et al. (1987b) showed a 3-year cumulative patency rate of 92% in the case of claudication and 79% limb salvage. Darling et al. (1993) reported a 5-year patency rate of 82%.

Aortoiliac Endarterectomy (Fig. 4)

Endarterectomy is a difficult technique, the indications for which have diminished since the development of transluminal angioplasty. It is mostly indicated in aortic and primitive iliac lesions. Endarterectomy of the EIA is less satisfactory (Naylor et al. 1990).

Direct endarterectomy is performed by proximal and distal clamping. The artery is opened longitudinally and the atheroma is

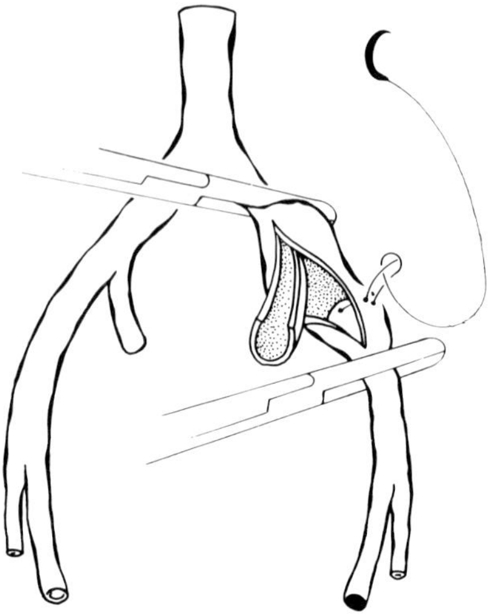

Fig. 4. Direct iliac endarterectomy: the artery is clamped, atheroma lifted, and distal external media sutured

lifted, dissected, and removed. Arteriotomy should extend beyond the site of the ablation of the atheroma in order to be able to control this point and to suture the distal external media to the wall. Distal control of the atheroma is often hazardous via the direct route at the level of the iliac bifurcation. Indirect endarterectomy is achieved by a transverse opening of the artery, lifting of the atheroma, and insertion of a loop stripper in proximal direction between the atheroma and the external part of the media. Proximally, a second transverse incision allows extraction of the material. The EIA can thus be handled blindly via a femoral approach. In the hands of an experienced surgeon, endarterectomy gives satisfactory results. The cumulative patency at 10 years is 80% for nonsmokers and 61% for smokers (Naylor et al. 1990).

Extra-anatomic Bypasses

Extra-anatomic bypasses permit revascularization of the lower limb when, due to the general condition of the partient, aortic clamping is not possible or when abdominal conditions do not favor vascular implantation (multiple postoperative status, infection, radiotherapy, tumor) (Rutherford et al. 1987). Extra-anatomic bypasses revascularizing the lower limb can be implanted distally on the

CFA, DFA, SFA, or the popliteal artery (PA). Only those bypasses terminating on the CFA are considered here as corresponding to the definition of DFA revascularization.

Axillobifemoral and Axillounifemoral Bypass (Fig. 5)

The axillobifemoral and axillounifemoral bypass is carried out by implantation of polyethylene terephtalate prosthesis or PTFE with an 8-mm diameter. This has an external framework, avoiding compression through the subcutaneous trunk and abdominal route. Proximal incision is subclavicular, usually on the right side (Blaisdell 1990). The pectoralis major is dissected and the first segment of the axillary artery is exposed. The femoral arteries are then prepared using the standard method. Proximal anastomosis is performed side-to-end using a 5–0 monofilament suture. The extra-anatomic path is laid out. It is preferable to pass the prosthesis under the external oblique and pectoralis major. A thoracic counterincision is usually required in order to produce an ideal curvature of the prosthesis. The horizontal branch of the bypass must not cross the abdomen subumbilically in an oblique fashion or take a recurrent route.

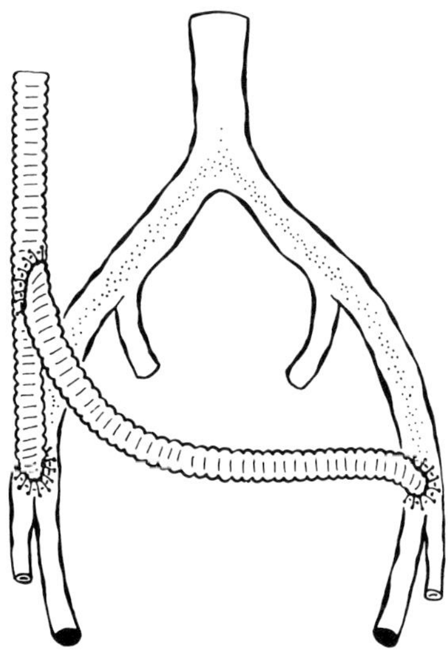

Fig. 5. Axillobifemoral bypass: the onset of the horizontal limb must be anticipated before performing proximal anastomosis

When a Y-prosthesis manufactured for this purpose is used, the length of the vertical limb and the onset of the horizontal one should be anticipated at the time of the proximal anastomosis. Distal anastomosis is carried out on the CFA using 5–0 monofilament suture. The horizontal limb is then passed subcutaneously or subfascially, and the heterolateral femoral anastomosis is performed. In general, axillobifemoral bypasses carry a more favorable prognosis than axillounifemoral bypasses (Lo Gerfo et al. 1977; Ward et al. 1983). Lo Gerfo et al. showed a 5-year patency rate of 74% for the former and 37% for the latter: the donor artery doubles its flow (Lo Gerfo et al. 1977; Shin and Chaudhry 1979; Ehrenfeld et al. 1968) and peripheral resistance falls (Dinis da Gama 1988) as the flow is distributed over several vascular peripheral beds. Long-term patency also depends upon the runoff and is better when the SFA is patent (Rutherford et al. 1987). Some authors, however, have been unable to confirm these findings both with regards to the point of view of patency between axillobifemoral and -unifemoral bypasses and with respect to the status of the peripheral circulation (Ascer et al. 1985). Finally, inflow into the bypass is important: if the donor artery is stenosed, it will be unable to adapt to the increase in flow. Therefore, supra-aortic preoperative angiography is indicated prior to axillofemoral bypass (Calligaro et al. 1990).

Femorofemoral Bypass (Fig. 6)

Femorofemoral bypass is indicated in unilateral iliac obstruction in the patient presenting with a significant surgical risk (Lee and Baird 1990). This technique avoids the opening of the peritoneal cavity, retroperitoneal dissection, and aortic clamping. Before considering femorofemoral bypass, however, one must consider the quality of the inflow. Indeed, the donor CFA flow must be normal without a pressure gradient detected with invasive measurement (Kalman et al. 1987a). The bypass will result in an iliac steal, and even with a normal donor iliac artery, a slight fall in postoperative pressure can be detected (Fahal et al. 1989).

Two inguinocrural incisions with exposure of the femoral arteries are performed. An end-to-side anastomosis is carried out between one CFA and a PTFE or Dacron 6- to 8-mm-diameter prosthesis. The anastomosis is performed using a 5–0 monofilament suture. It is advisable to give a slight S curvature to the bypass, taking the flow as high as possible on the CFA on the donor side and terminating on the distal CFA on the recipient side

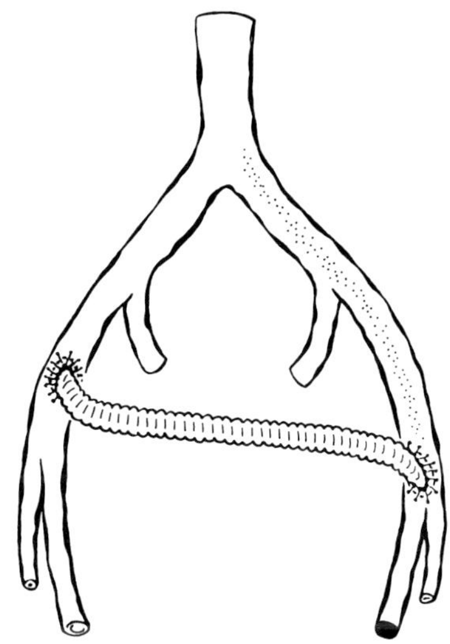

Fig. 6. Femorofemoral bypass: the prosthesis has a slight S curvature. Proximal anastomosis on the proximal common femoral artery (CFA) and distal anastomosis on the distal CFA

(Fahal et al. 1989; Perler et al. 1991). In order to accentuate the obliqueness of this pathway, the proximal anastomosis can be placed out on the EIA after a retroperitoneal exposure. Patency of the femorofemoral bypasses is from 80% to more than 90% at 1 year, between 60% and 80% at 5 years, and 60% at 10 years (Dick et al. 1980; Farber et al. 1990; Lamberton et al. 1985; Plecha and Plecha 1984). Patency is greater if the SFA is patent (Dick et al. 1980; Farber et al. 1990). Perler et al. (1991), however, reported less favorable results for femorofemoral bypass than for the iliofemoral bypass: 5-year patency rate of 57% in the former and 93% in the latter.

Thoracofemoral Bypass (Fig. 7)

Although first described in 1961 (Stevenson et al. 1961; Blaisdell et al. 1961), thoracofemoral bypass has not been widely performed until recent years. For a long period of time, axillofemoral bypass was preferred. However, the popularity of thoracofemoral bypass is growing, due to its satisfactory results. Nevertheless, it is not indicated as a first-line treatment, but should be considered after obstruction of an aorto- or axillofemoral bypass, in the case of

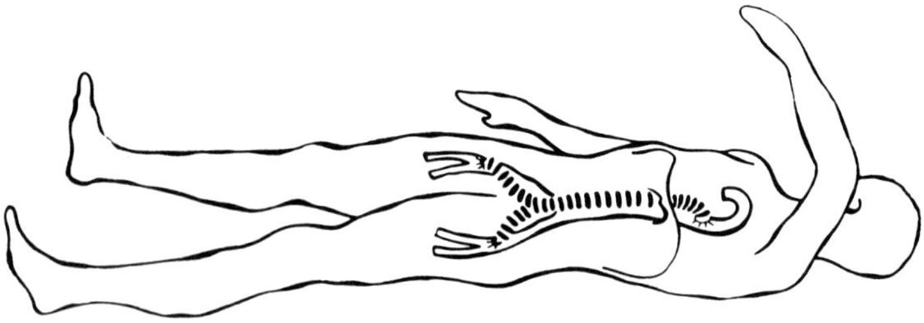

Fig. 7. Thoracofemoral bypass: the pelvis is flat and left hemithorax slightly lifted up

abdominal infection, in the presence of a highly calcified aorta, or in the presence of major intraperitoneal adhesions.

The patient is placed with the pelvis flat and the left hemithorax at 45°. The femoral arteries are dissected. The left inguinal incision can be extended proximally in order to retract the abdominal muscle and prepare the retroperitoneal route for the prosthesis (Criado et al. 1992). An oblique incision of the left flank with retraction of the muscles of the abdominal wall enables the retroperitoneal path to be completed behind the left kidney to the diaphragm as far as the left costodiaphragmatic sinus. A lateral thoracotomy is performed in the seventh intercostal space. The left lung is collapsed and the line of pleural reflection is incised. The aorta is carefully surrounded and tangentially clamped. A Y-shaped Dacron or PTFE prosthesis is beveled and anastomosed in an end-to-side position using a 3–0 monofilament suture. The prosthesis is passed from the thorax to the retroperitoneum and anastomosis between the left limb and the CFA is then carried out using 4–0 or 5–0 monofilament suture. The right limb is passed subfascially and the right end-to-side anastomosis performed.

This technique produces a better inflow than an axillofemoral bypass. Moreover, the main branch of the prosthesis lies within the body cavities and is thus protected from external compression. Surgical mortality is less than 10% and long-term patency is better than for axillofemoral bypasses, at approximately 70% (Branchereau et al. 1992).

Transluminal Angioplasty (Fig. 8)

Aortoiliac transluminal angioplasty should also be considered as a method for DFA revascularization. Although it does not entail surgical revascularization at the ostium, such as an anastomosis on the CFA, it improves flow at the takeoff of the DFA by removing a stenosis or an obstruction. Angioplasty, developed by Dotter and Judkins (1964), often replaces traditional revascularization. This technique has expanded rapidly and is not only applicable to the aortoiliac segment, but also to the femoropopliteal and crural arteries and also to the DFA. It is in the aortoiliac region that it is of interest in this chapter and this is also where it produces its best results.

Transluminal angioplasty is currently used by radiologists and cardiologists. It also constitutes part of the armamen tarium of vascular surgeons (Veith et al. 1991) who know the indication for revascularization and who can immediately convert an angioplasty failure and combine a proximal angioplasty to a peripheral bypass or, alternatively, can dilate peripheral stenotic lesions during a proximal bypass. The technique is well described in renowned publications (Mahler 1990). The CFA is punctured using Seldinger technique and a 35-cm guide is inserted in a proximal direction. An

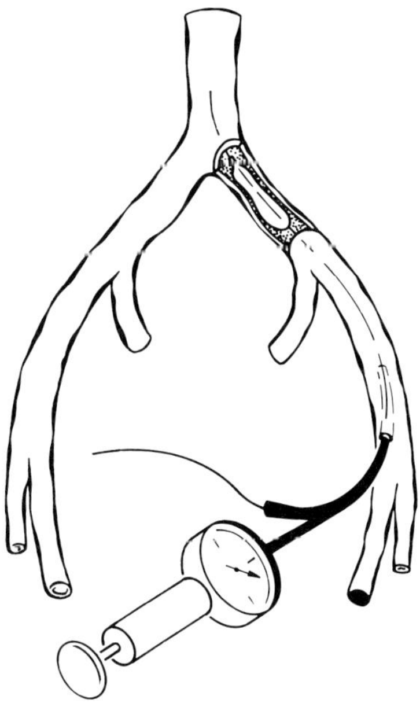

Fig. 8. Transluminal angioplasty: dilation of an internal iliac stenosis under manometric control

introducer is passed along the guiding wire and enters the iliac artery, distal to the stenosis. Using a lateral connection, it is possible to measure the distal blood pressure. The short guiding wire is then removed and replaced by a longer J-guide (150 cm) and is passed beyond the stenosis. It is introduced under radioscopic control as far as the distal aorta. The dilatation catheter is then placed onto the guide via the introducer. The balloon is placed at the level of the stenosis and dilatation is carried out under manometric and radioscopic control. After dilatation, angiography with pressure measurement is performed.

Ideally, transluminal dilatation is indicated in the case of a short and symptomatic stenosis of the aortoiliac segment. The indications have expanded with the development of the method and currently include long stenoses and obstructions. Likewise, angioplasty was first indicated for patients in a poor general condition in a situation of limb salvage who were unable to tolerate conventional surgery. Angioplasty can now be undertaken for lesions only producing a moderate claudication. However, it would appear reasonable not to go on to treat radiologic stenoses without hemodynamic significance, and preoperative evaluation – especially duplex scanning – is recommended (Vashisht et al. 1992).

Aortoiliac dilatation is a very effective method. More than 90% of lesions can be dilated with success and the morbidity is less than 10%. The 5-year patency rate varies from 53% to 85% (Johnston 1992; Tegtmeyer et al. 1991). Good prognostic factors include stenosis (rather than an obstruction), a lesion affecting the primitive iliac artery (rather than disease of the EIA), angioplasty for claudication (rather than limb salvage), and a well-developed peripheral circulation.

Iliac angioplasty can be carried out alone or associated with the insertion of a stent. As in the case of angioplasty alone, it is at this level that the results are best. Indications for stents are dissection induced by angioplasty, a recurrence of stenosis after the first angioplasty, an inadequate angioplasty with persistence of a 30% stenosis, and a transstenotic pressure gradient greater than 5 mmHg (Becker 1991; Palmaz et al. 1990).

What are the Choices After Deep Femoral Artery Revascularization? (Fig. 9)

Revascularization aims at increasing the flow at the entrance of the DFA in the case of proximal stenosis or obstruction. Strictly speaking, in revascularization, a procedure associated with the DFA or a femoropopliteal bypass is not performed because it is impossible or not indicated.

However, revascularization can, in certain circumstances, be associated with a specific procedure on the DFA – profundaplasty (Chap. 9), reconstruction (Chap. 10), or a femoropopliteal bypass – when it appears to be insufficient to treat a severe claudication or to save a limb. Indications for combining peripheral surgery with aortoiliac revascularization are discussed in Chaps. 6 and 9, i.e., a two-level disease in a condition of limb salvage. The recovery of a pulsed flow to the peripheral level offers the best chance of stopping the development of necrosis.

After revascularization, profundaplasty (or reconstruction) can be added. The indication is a two-level disease associated with DFA disease. Two conditions must be present for this option to be selected: the first is the impossibility of carrying out a femoropopliteal bypass, usually due to inadequate runoff; the second is a patent distal DFA. Profundaplasty or reconstruction is performed on the proximal DFA according to the indications discussed in Chaps. 9 and 10 (profundaplasty in the case of stenosis, reconstruction in the event of obstruction).

After revascularization, profundaplasty and femoropopliteal bypass can also be undertaken. The indication is also a two-level disease. This option is chosen when three conditions are met: a patent distal DFA, a good collateral network between the DFA and the PA (profundapopliteal collateral index, PPCI < 0.2), and a good PA runoff, enabling femoropopliteal bypass.

Finally, after revascularization, a femoropopliteal bypass alone, without DFA intervention, can be carried out. The indication is

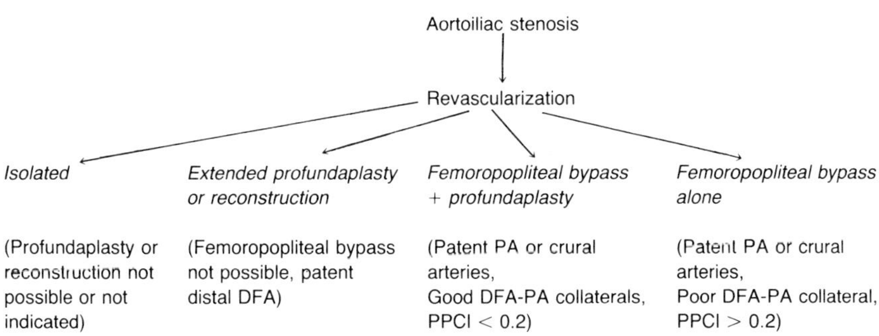

Fig. 9. Possibilities after deep femoral artery (DFA) revascularization. *PA*, popliteal artery; *PPCI*, profundapopliteal collateral index

still a two-level disease. This option is chosen when the collateral network between DFA and PA is inadequate (PPCI > 0.2), but when a good PA runoff is present.

References

Ascer E, Veith FJ, Gupta SK, Scher LA, Samson RH, White-Flores SA, Sprayregen S (1985) Comparison of axillounifemoral and axillobifemoral bypass operations. Surgery 97: 169–175

Bagi P, Sillesen H, Hansen HJB (1988) Quantitative Doppler ultrasound evaluation of occlusive arterial disease in the lower limb. Eur J Vasc Surg 2: 409–415

Bagi P, Sillesen H, Bitsch K, Hansen HJB (1990) Doppler waveform analysis in evaluation of occlusive arterial disease in the lower limb: comparison with distal blood pressure measurement and arteriography. Eur J Vasc Surg 4: 305–311

Baker JD (1990) Hemodynamic assessment of aortoiliac segment. Surg Clin North Am 70: 31–40

Barringer M, Poole GV, Shircliffe AC, Meredith JW, Hightower F, Plonk GW (1983) The diagnosis of aortoiliac disease. A noninvasive femoral cuff technique. Ann Surg 197: 204–209

Becker GJ (1991) Intravascular stents. General principles and status of lower-extremity arterial applications. Circulation 83 [Suppl I]: I-122–I-136

Bernhard VM, Ray LI, Militello JP (1976) The role of angioplasty of the profunda femoris artery in revascularization of the ischemic limb. Surg Gynecol Obstet 142: 840–844

Bettmann MA (1992) Principles of angiography. In: Loscalzo J, Creager MA, Dzau VJ (eds) Vascular medicine. Little and Brown, Boston, pp 483–507

Blaisdell FW (1990) Axillofemoral and axillopopliteal grafts. In: Bergan JJ, Yao JST (eds) Techniques in vascular surgery. Saunders, Philadelphia, pp 339–348

Blaisdell FW, DeMattei GA, Gauder PJ (1961) Extraperitoneal aorta to femoral bypass graft as replacement for an infected aortic bifurcation prosthesis. Am J Surg 102: 583–585

Branchereau A, Magnan PE, Moracchini P, Espinoza H, Mathieu JP (1992) Use of descending thoracic aorta for lower limb revascularization. Eur J Vasc Surg 6: 255–262

Calligaro KD, Ascer E, Veith FJ, Gupta SK, Wengerter KR, Franco CD, Bakal CW, Sprayregen S (1990) Unsuspected inflow disease in candidates for axillofemoral bypass operations: a prospective study. J Vasc Surg 11: 832–837

Carpenter JP, Owen RS, Baum RA, Cope C, Barker CF, Berkowitz HD, Golden MA, Perloff LJ (1992) Magnetic resonance angiography of peripheral runoff vessels. J Vasc Surg 16: 807–815

Cossman DV, Ellison JE, Wagner WH, Carroll RM, Treiman RL, Foran RF, Levin PM, Cohen JL (1989) Comparison of contrast arteriography to arterial mapping with color-flow duplex imaging in the lower extremities. J Vasc Surg 10: 522–529

Criado E, Johnson G Jr, Burnham SJ, Buehrer J, Keagy BA (1992) Descending thoracic aorta-to-iliofemoral artery bypass as an alternative to aortoiliac reconstruction. J Vasc Surg 15: 550–557

Darling RC III, Leather RP, Chang BB, Lloyd WE, Shah DM (1993) Is iliac artery a suitable inflow conduit for iliofemoral occlusive disease: an analysis of 514 aortoiliac reconstructions. J Vasc Surg 17: 15–22

Dick LS, Brief DK, Alpert J, Brener BJ, Goldenkranz R, Parsonnet V (1980) A 12-year experience with femorofemoral crossover grafts. Arch Surg 115: 1359–1365

Dietzek AM, Goldsmith J, Veith FJ, Sanchez LA, Gupta SK, Wengerter KR (1990) Interruption of critical aortoiliac collateral circulation during nonvascular operations: a cause of acute limb-threatening ischemia. J Vasc Surg 12: 645–653

Dinis da Gama A (1988) The fate of donor artery in extraanatomic revascularization. J Vasc Surg 8: 106–111

Dotter CT, Judkins MP (1964) Transluminal treatment of arteriosclerotic obstruction: description of a new technic and a preliminary report of its application. Circulation 30: 654–670

Edwards WH, Jenkins JM, Muhlherin JL, Martin RS, Edwards WH Jr (1989) Extended profundoplasty to minimize pelvic and distal tissue loss. Ann Surg 211: 694–702

Ehrenfeld WK, Harris JD, Wylie EJ (1968) Vascular "steal" phenomenon. An experimental study. Am J Surg 116: 192–197

Fahal AH, McDonald AM, Marston A (1989) Femorofemoral bypass in unilateral iliac artery occlusion. Br J Surg 76: 22–25

Farber MA, Hollier LH, Eubanks R, Ochsner JL, Bowen JC (1990) Femorofemoral bypass: a profile of graft failure. South Med J 83: 1437–1443

Feldhaus RJ, Sterpetti AV, Schultz RD, Peetz DJ (1985) A technique for profunda femoris artery reconstruction. Ann Surg 203: 390–398

Flanigan DP, Ryan TJ, Williams LR, Schwartz JA, Gray B, Schuler JJ (1984) Aortofemoral or femoropopliteal revascularization? A prospective evaluation of the papaverine test. J Vasc Surg 1: 215–223

Friedenberg MJ, Perez CA (1965) Collateral circulation in aorto-ilio-femoral occlusive disease. Am J Roentgenol 94: 145–158

Gaylis H (1992) Interruption of critical aortoiliac circulation during nonvascular operations: a cause of acute limb-threatening ischemia. J Vasc Surg 15: 256–257

Goldstone J (1990) Management of late failures of aorto-femoral reconstructions. Acta Chir Scand Suppl 555: 149–153

Guidoin R, King M, Deng X, Paris E, Douville Y (1992) Prothèses artérielles en polyester. In: Kieffer E (ed) Le remplacement artériel: principes et applications. AERCV, Paris, pp 3–51

Gupta SK, Veith FJ, Kram HB, Wengerter KA (1990) Significance and management of inflow gradients unexpectedly generated after femorofemoral, femoropopliteal, and femoroinfrapopliteal bypass grafting. J Vasc Surg 12: 278–283

Iliopoulos JI, Pierce GE, McCroskey BL, Thomas JH, Hermreck AS (1985) Success of profundoplasty: the role of the extent of deep femoral artery disease. Am J Surg 150: 753–756

Iliopoulos JI, Hermreck AS, Thomas JH, Pierce GE (1989) Hemodynamics of the hypogastric arterial circulation. J Vasc Surg 9: 637–642

Iliopoulos JI, Pierce GE, Hermreck AS, Haller CC, Thomas JH (1990) Hemodynamics of the inferior mesenteric arterial circulation. J Vasc Surg 11: 120–126

Jausseran JM, Nazet J, Chbib A, Bergeron P, Rudondy P, Ferdani M, Courbier R (1991) Revascularisation de l'artère fémorale profonde distale. J Chir 128: 26–29

Johnston KW (1987) Peripheral arterial Doppler blood flow velocity waveform analysis. In: Kempczinski RF, Yao JST (eds) Practical noninvasive vascular diagnosis. Year Book Medical Publishers, Chicago, pp 154–177

Johnston KW (1990) Aortoiliac reconstruction. In: Barnes RW (ed) Peripheral vascular surgery. American College of Surgeons, San Francisco, pp 7–9

Johnston KW (1992) Factors that influence the outcome of aortoiliac and femoropopliteal percutaneous transluminal angioplasty. Surg Clin North Am 72: 843–850

Kalman PG, Hosang M, Johnston KW, Walker PM (1987a) The current role for femorofemoral bypass. J Vasc Surg 6: 71–76

Kalman PG, Hosang M, Johnston KW, Walker PM (1987b) Unilateral iliac disease: the role of iliofemoral bypass. J Vasc Surg 6: 139–143

Kitslaar PJEHM, Jörning PJG, Köhlen JPFM (1988) Assessment of aortoiliac stenosis by femoral artery pressure measurement and Doppler waveform analysis. Eur J Vac Surg 2: 35–40

Kohler TP, Nance DR, Cramer MM, Vandenburge N, Strandness DE Jr (1987) Duplex scanning for diagnosis of aortoiliac and femoropopliteal disease: a prospective study. Circulation 76: 1074–1080

Krahl E, Pratt GH, Rousselot LM, Ruzicka FF (1954) The collateral circulation in the arterial occlusive disease of the lower extremity. Surg Gynecol Obstet 98: 320–324

Kram HB, Gupta SK, Veith FJ, Wengerter KR (1991) Unilateral aortofemoral bypass: a safe and effective option for the treatment of unilateral limb-threatening ischemia. Am J Surg 162: 155–158

Krupski WC, Sumchai A, Effeney DJ, Ehrenfeld WK (1984) The importance of abdominal wall collateral blood vessels. Arch Surg 119: 854–857

Lamberton AJ, Nicolaides AN, Eastcott HHG (1985) The femorofemoral graft. Arch Surg 120: 1274–1278

Lee RE, Baird RN (1990) A haemodynamic evaluation of the femoro-femoral cross-over bypass. Eur J Vasc Surg 4: 167–172

Legemate DA, Ackerstaff RGA, Eikelboom BC (1989) Duplex scanning in cerebral, abdominal and peripheral arterial disease. Eur J Vasc Surg 3: 287–295

Legemate DA, Teeuwen C, Hoeneveld H, Eikelboom BC (1991) Value of duplex scanning compared with angiography and pressure measurement in the assessment of aortoiliac arterial lesions. Br J Surg 78: 1003–1008

Lo Gerfo FW, Johnson WC, Corson JD, Vollman RW, Weisel RD, Davis RC, O'Hara ET, Nasbeth DC, Mannick JA (1977) A comparison of the late patency rates of axillobilateral femoral and axillounilateral femoral grafts. Surgery 81: 33–38

Lorentzen JE, Jørgensen L, Johansen JJ (1990) The ideal operation for unilateral iliac occlusion. Should the asymptomatic iliac artery also be reconstructed? Acta Chir Scand Suppl 555: 69–71

Mahler F (1990) PTA der Beckenarterien und terminalen Aorta. In: Mahler F (ed) Katheterinterventionen in der Angiologie. Thieme, Stuttgart, pp 79–131

McCoy DM, Sawchuk AP, Schuler JJ, Durham JR, Eldrup-Jorgensen J, Schwarcz TH, Meyer JP, Flanigan P (1989) The role of isolated profundaplasty for the treatment of rest pain. Arch Surg 124: 441–444

Mellière D, Labastie J, Becquemin JP, Kassab M, Paris E (1990) Proximal anastomosis in aortobifemoral bypass: end-to-end or end-to-side ? J Cardiovasc Surg 31: 77–80

Miksic K, Novak B (1986) Profunda femoris revascularization in limb salvage. J Cardiovasc Surg 27: 544–552

Naylor AR, Ah-See AK, Engeset J (1990) Aortoiliac endarterectomy: an 11-year review. Br J Surg 77: 190–193

Nunez AA, Veith FJ, Collier P, Ascer E, White-Flores SA, Gupta SK (1988) Direct approaches to the distal portions of the deep femoral artery for limb salvage bypasses. J Vasc Surg 8: 576–581

Ouriel K, De Weese JA, Ricotta JJ, Green RM (1987) Revascularization of the distal profunda femoris artery in the reconstructive treatment of aortoiliac occlusive disease. J Vasc Surg 6: 217–220

Paes EHJ, Hamann H (1989) Die Profundarevaskularisation: eine vergessene Alternative zur Mehretagenrekonstruktion. Vasa 18: 287–290

Palmaz JC, Garcia OJ, Shatz RA, Rees CR, Roeren T, Richter GM, Noeldge G, Gardiner GA, Becker GJ, Walker C, Stagg J, Katzen BT, Dake MD, Paolini RM, McLean GK, Lammer J, Schwarten DE, Tio FO, Root HD, Rogers W (1990) Placement of balloon-expandable intraluminal stents in iliac arteries: first 171 procedures. Radiology 174: 969–975

Perler BA, Burdick JF, Williams GM (1991) Femoro-femoral or ilio-femoral bypass for unilateral inflow reconstruction? Am J Surg 161: 426–430

Persson AV, Gibbons G, Griffey S (1981) Noninvasive evaluation of the aortoiliac segment. J Cardiovasc Surg 22: 539–542

Piotrowski JJ, Pearce WH, Jones DN, Whitehill T, Bell R, Patt, Rutherford RB (1988) Aortobifemoral bypass: the operation of choice for unilateral iliac occlusion? J Vasc Surg 8: 211 –218

Plecha FR, Plecha FM (1984) Femorofemoral bypass grafts: ten-year experience. J Vasc Surg 1: 555–561

Rollins DL, Towne JB, Bernhard VM, Baum PL (1985) Isolated profundaplasty for limb salvage. J Vasc Surg 2: 585–590

Rutherford RB, Patt A, Pearce WH (1987) Extra-anatomic bypass: a closer review. J Vasc Surg 6: 437–446

Sawchuk AP, Flanigan P, Tober JC, Eton D, Schwarcz TH, Eldrup-Jorgensen J, Meyer JP, Durham JR, Schuler JJ (1990) A rapid, accurate, noninvasive technique for diagnosing critical and subcritical stenoses in aortoiliac arteries. J Vasc Surg 12: 158–167

Schwilden ED, van Dongen RJAM (1987) Eingriffe an der Arteria profunda femoris. In: Heberer G, van Dongen RJAM (eds) Gefässchirurgie. Springer, Berlin Heidelberg New York, pp 457–473

Shin CS, Chaudhry AG (1979) The hemodynamics of extra-anatomic bypass grafts. Surg Gynecol Obstet 148: 567–570

Stevenson JK, Sauvage LR, Harkins HN (1961) A bypass homograft from thoracic aorta to femoral arteries for occlusive vascular disease. Case report. Am Surg 27: 632–637

Sumner DS (1989) Essential hemodynamic principles. In: Rutherford RB (ed) Vascular surgery. Saunders, Philadelphia, pp 18–41

Szilagyi DE, Elliot JP, Smith RF, Reddy DJ, McPharlin M (1986) A thirty-year survey of the reconstructive surgical treatment of aortoiliac occlusive disease. J Vasc Surg 3: 421–436

Tegtmeyer CJ, Hartwell GD, Selby JB, Robertson R Jr, Kron IL, Tribble CG (1991) Results and complications of angioplasty in aortoiliac disease. Circulation 83 [Suppl I]: I-53–I-60

Towne JB, Rollins DL (1986) Profundaplasty: its role in limb salvage. Surg Clin North Am 66: 403–414

van der Heijden FHWM, Legemate DA, van Leeuwen MS, Mali WPTM, Eikelboom BC (1993) Value of duplex scanning in the selection of patients for percutaneous transluminal angioplasty. Eur J Vasc Surg 7: 71–76

Vashisht R, Ellis MR, Skidmore C, Blair SD, Greenhalgh RM, O'Malley MK (1992) Colour-coded duplex ultrasonography in the selection of patients for endovascular surgery. Br J Surg 79: 1030–1031

Veith FJ, Gupta SK, Wengerter KR, Rivers SP, Bakal CW (1991) Impact of nonoperative therapy on the clinical management of peripheral arterial disease. Circulation 83 [Suppl I]: I-137–I-142

Ward RE, Holcroft JW, Conti S, Blaisdell FW (1983) New concepts in the use of axillofemoral bypass grafts. Arch Surg 118: 573–576

9 Profundaplasty

R.J.A.M. van Dongen

Definition and Terminology

A profundaplasty must be distinguished from other operative procedures performed on the deep femoral artery (DFA). The confusing terminology in this field makes a clear definition necessary.

A profundaplasty (called by some authors "isolated profondaplasty") is a surgical procedure performed on the takeoff, the proximal part, and the trunk of the DFA with the intention of maximizing blood flow through the DFA and the profundapopliteal collaterals by eliminating anatomical, hemodynamic, geometric, and pathological hitches, obstructions, and resistance. A profundaplasty can be considered in patients with an occluded superficial femoral artery (SFA) and unimpaired iliac and common femoral arterial (CFA) flow.

The term "profunda revascularization" (Chap. 8) should be reserved for procedures which improve or restore pulsatile blood flow to the proximal portion of the unimpaired DFA in patients with two-level (pelvic and femoropopliteal) occlusive disease. In fact, it concerns methods which restore blood flow through the iliac artery and the CFA to the unobstructed DFA. A mere profunda revascularization does not include surgical procedures on the DFA itself. However, to improve runoff conditions, a DFA revascularization should always be combined with a profundaplasty.

The term "profunda reconstruction" (Chap. 10) should be reserved exclusively for reconstructive procedures performed on a totally occluded or arteriosclerotically narrowed DFA trunk in patients with femoropopliteal occlusive disease. In most such cases the distal bifurcation of the DFA will remain unimpaired, so that the DFA itself can be treated successfully with endarterectomy and patch graft, replaced by an interposition graft, or bridged with a bypass graft. Sometimes the inflow tract will also be affected by arteriosclerosis. In such cases, DFA reconstruction must be combined with DFA revascularization.

Anatomical, Pathologic, Hemodynamic, and Geometric Aspects

Under normal circumstances the DFA provides the blood supply to the muscles of the thigh, and the SFA transports blood to the knee region, the lower leg, and the foot. However, when degenerative disease obstructs the SFA, the DFA enlarges and together with the profundapopliteal collateral system becomes a most efficient alternative conduit, transporting blood from the CFA to the popliteal artery (PA). The feasibility of utilizing the collateral circulation of the DFA for revascularization of the lower extremity was described in 1961 by Leeds and Gilfillan and by Morris et al. (1961).

The DFA and its collaterals can take over the function of the SFA to a great extent. Unfortunately, the condition of the origin and trunk of the DFA does not allow full utilization of the potential capacity of the profundapopliteal collateral bed. Optimal blood flow through the DFA is impeded by four obstacles.

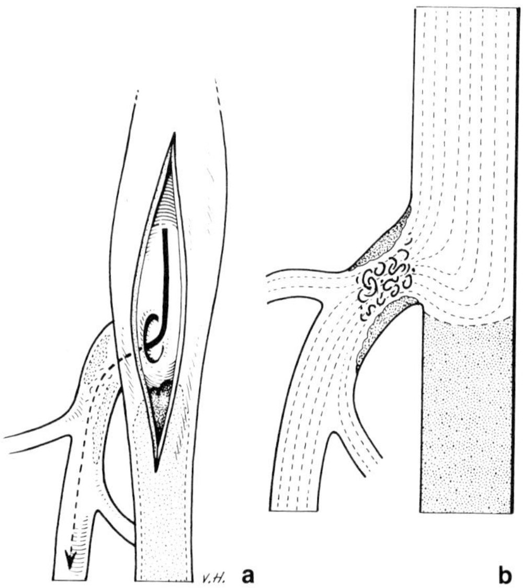

Fig. 1. a The dorsolateral takeoff of the deep femoral artery (DFA) causes a hemodynamically unfavorable kink in the blood flow when the superficial femoral artery (SFA) is occluded. Narrowing of the proximal portion of the DFA caused by thickening of the arterial wall with plaque formation. **b** Turbulences in the proximal portion of the DFA, caused by kinking of the blood flow, abrupt reduction in vessel caliber, intimal thickening, and wall irregularities

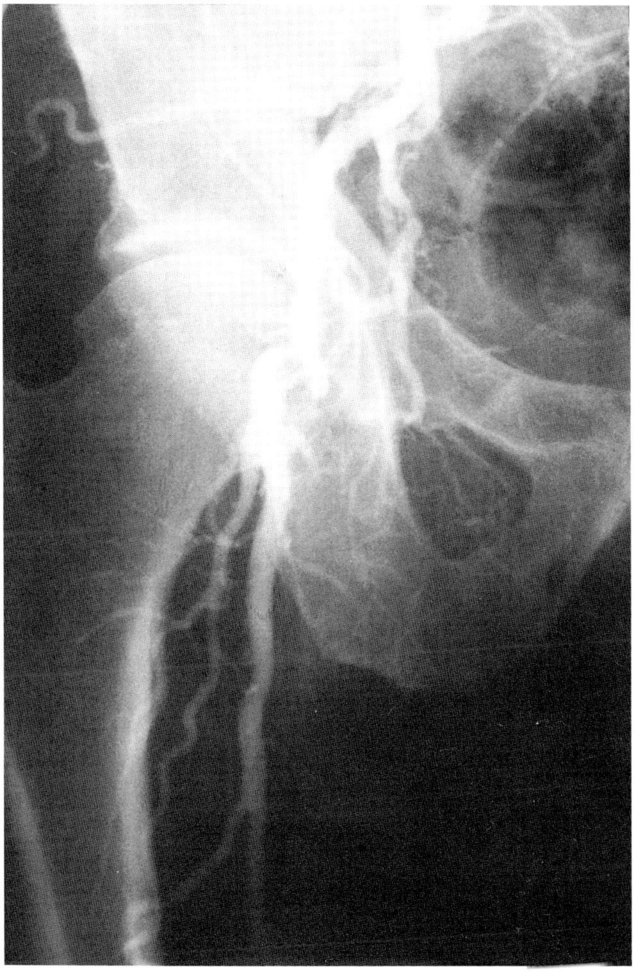

Fig. 2. Kinking of the conduit and arteriosclerotic narrowing of the proximal portion of the deep femoral artery (DFA) are best seen when arteriograms are made with the patient in the oblique position

The origin of the DFA is the first weak point. The kink in the conduit formed by the dorsolateral takeoff of the DFA causes considerable loss of kinetic energy and therefore decreased blood flow (Figs. 1a, 2). This is a *hemodynamic* obstacle.

The proximal portion of the DFA often shows arteriosclerotic narrowing caused by thickening of the arterial wall and plaque formation, especially in the presence of femoropopliteal occlusion. The true incidence and the extent of these lesions are more clearly appreciated when angiograms in oblique views are obtained (Fig.

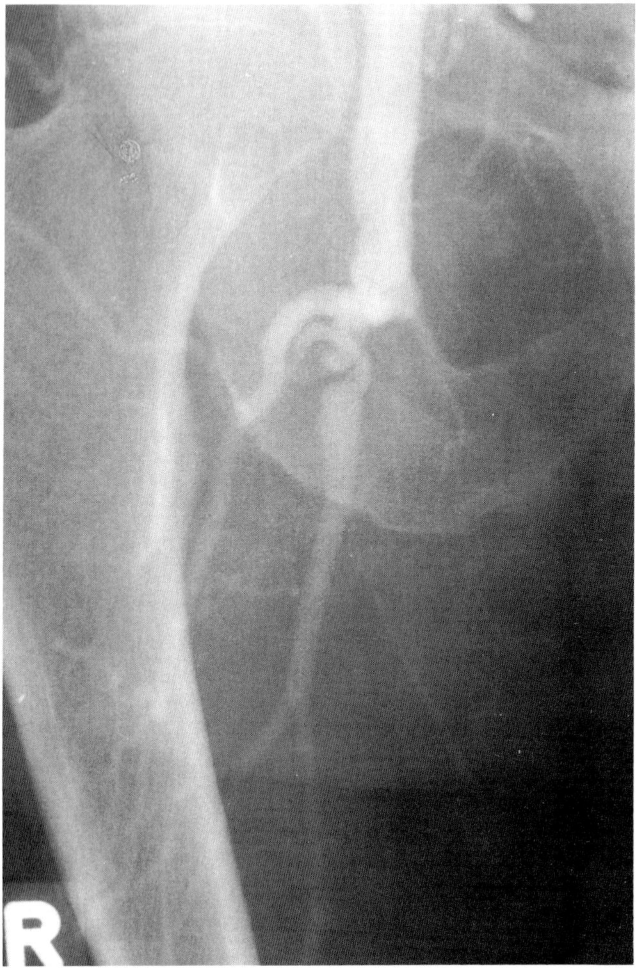

Fig. 3. Arteriosclerotic irregularities and narrowing in the proximal portion of the deep femoral artery (DFA)

3). Beales et al. (1971) noted narrowing of the DFA in 59% of patients with femoropopliteal occlusion. In 74% of affected limbs, narrowing was localized in the proximal portion of the DFA and extended into the trunk for a short distance. This is a *pathological* obstacle, an organic stenosis.

A third obstruction is formed by *turbulence* of blood flow in the proximal portion of the DFA (Fig. 1b). This turbulence is caused by kinking of blood flow at the origin of the DFA, abrupt reduction in vessel caliber at the transition of the CFA into the DFA, intimal thickening of the proximal DFA, and irregularities

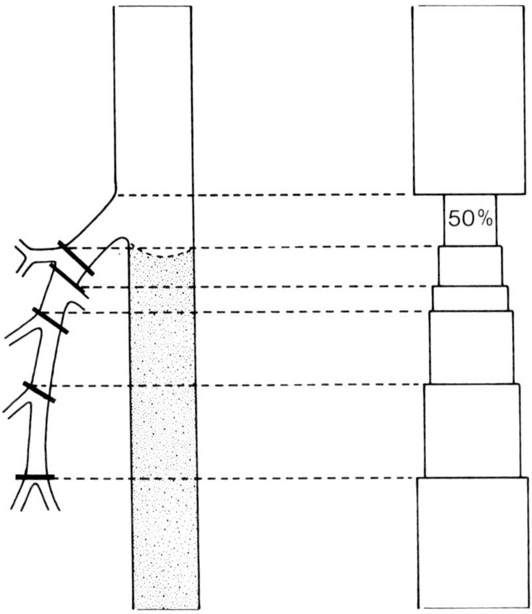

Fig. 4. Occlusion of the superficial femoral artery (SFA), effectively causing the deep femoral artery (DFA) to act as an area of stenosis. Progressive increase in cross-sectional area at successive divisions beyond the common femoral artery (CFA) due to the effect of the bifurcation area ratio

at the site of the SFA origin. All this turbulence causes further reduction of blood flow; it acts as a stenosis.

The *geometric* condition of the DFA trunk forms a fourth impediment for maximal blood flow. Investigations and geometric analyses by Berguer et al. (1975b) define the importance of this factor as cause of reduced blood flow through the DFA.

At any major arterial bifurcation, including the femoral bifurcation, the total cross-sectional area of the branches is greater than that of the common trunk. When the SFA is occluded, the flow tract undergoes an abrupt reduction in caliber at the level of the origin of the DFA. Berguer et al. (1975a) demonstrated that the mean value of the area ratio (i.e., the cross-sectional area of the DFA divided by the area of the CFA) is equal to 0.5. That means that, independently of existing wall lesions within the DFA, the proximal portion of the DFA itself represents an anatomical stenosis of about 50% (Fig. 4). From the level of the origins of the femoral circumflex arteries, the DFA divides many times along a short distance. At each arterial division, the total cross-sectional area increases. Thus, in accordance with the geometric principle, the proximal stenosis will be relieved little by little at the level of each division. Not until the most distal branching has been reached will the stenosis of the trunk be totally relieved. The entire trunk of the DFA acts as a geometric or anatomical stenosis.

Arteriosclerotic thickening of the DFA wall is one of the factors contributing to the degree of stenosis, and of course this in turn has significant negative influence on blood flow. However, removal of arteriosclerotic material alone will not bring about sufficient hemodynamic improvement. The geometric stenosis of the DFA, interposed between the CFA and the profundapopliteal collateral system, must be relieved as well. This can be achieved by enlargement of the DFA over its entire length. To obtain a maximal effect the enlargement must be extended down to the most distal perforating artery (Leather et al. 1978; Lawson et al. 1983; Taylor et al. 1981; David and Drezner 1978; Schwilden and van Dongen 1989).

Aims and Requirements of an Efficient Profundaplasty

The purpose of a profundaplasty is to obtain an optimal utilization of the capacity of the profundapopliteal collateral system. This aim will be achieved when all morphologic and hemodynamic obstacles are eliminated:

1. The kinking of the blood flow at the origin of the DFA must be eliminated to obtain better hemodynamic conditions at the takeoff.
2. The pathologic arteriosclerotic stenosis of the proximal part of the DFA should be abolished by removing the thickening of the wall combined with (venous) patch grafting.
3. All sources of turbulence must be cleared away. The turbulent flow at the origin of the DFA must be changed into a laminar flow. The difference in diameter or cross-sectional area between the CFA and DFA can be eliminated by patch grafting. When the arteriosclerotic plaques in the proximal portion of the DFA are removed, this source of turbulence will disappear. The origin of the SFA is another source of turbulence which should be removed.
4. It is important to eliminate the geometric stenosis of the DFA by enlarging this vessel as far distally as possible. Reestablishing adequate flow to all branches of the DFA is vital to the success of the operation. Limiting the enlargement procedure to the proximal portion of the DFA or to the diseased area alone, without inclusion of the rest of the trunk with its geometrically

significant branches, is inadequate from a hemodynamic point of view. It merely lessens, but does not relieve, the preexisting anatomical stenosis.

Not until all these conditions are fulfilled can the potential capacity of the DFA and the profundapopliteal collateral circuit be completely utilized.

Indications

It is generally accepted that reconstructive vascular surgery should be reserved for patients who are unable to continue their work or are incapacitated in their daily life activities. Only patients with rest pain, progressing necrosis, or incapacitating claudication are candidates for surgery. This is not usually indicated for uncomplicated arterial occlusion with mild to moderate claudication, since the prognosis for such lesions is generally favorable if adequate conservative treatment is attempted. This also applies to the use of profundaplasty. Ninety percent of our patients subjected to profundaplasty had rest pain, distal necrosis, or a walking ability of less than 100 m. Exceptions have been made for patients needing a longer walking capacity for professional or social reasons.

A profundaplasty aims at compensating for the occlusion of the SFA via the collateral system of the thigh (Martin and Jamieson 1974). The effectiveness of this operation depends not only upon the technical and hemodynamic perfection of the procedure, but also to a great extent on the condition of the DFA and on the number and condition of preexisting profundapopliteal collaterals and their entry sites. Moreover, the quality of the collateral recipient segment of the PA, the PA itself, and the lower leg arteries is very important (Boren et al. 1980; Strandness, 1970). In many cases the question arises as to whether a profundaplasty will be an adequate procedure to cure the ischemic symptoms of the limb or whether a femoropopliteal or femorocrural bypass operation should be preferred. Table 1 provides useful guidelines for selection of the operations in patients with femoral occlusion and unimpaired aortoiliac inflow.

In patients with (a) angiographically demonstrated stenosis of the proximal DFA, (b) numerous and wide profundapopliteal collaterals, (c) an undiseased or only slightly arteriosclerotic recipient segment of the PA, and (d) good condition of the PA and lower leg arteries, circumstances are ideal for profundaplasty and a significant improvement of ischemic symptoms can be expected

Table 1. Factors influencing the choice between profundaplasty and femorodistal bypass operation in patients with occluded superficial femoral artery (SFA) and unimpaired inflow tract

DFA	Criteria			
	Potential capacity of profundapopliteal collateral system (PPCI)	Quality of collateral entry sites and PA recipient segment	Quality of PA and lower leg arteries	Procedure of choice
Proximal stenosis	Good (PPCI < 0.25)	Good	Good	Profundaplasty
Without stenosis	Poor (PPCI > 0.5)	Poor	Good	Femorodistal bypass
Without stenosis	Poor (PPCI > 0.5)	Poor	Poor	Femorodistal bypass or profundaplasty dependent on factors listed in "Indications"

DFA, deep femoral artery; PA, popliteal artery

(Myhre 1977; Watelet et al. 1978; Schwilden and van Dongen 1989). Because of the relatively short operation time required, the technical simplicity of the procedure, and the favorable long-term prognosis, profundaplasty should be preferred to femoropopliteal bypass under these circumstances. Only the social or professional requirement of unrestricted walking capability favors a bypass procedures.

In the case of (a) a freely patent DFA, (b) insufficient profundapopliteal collateral circulation, and/or (c) stenoses of collateral entry sites or a significantly diseased collateral recipient segment of the PA, profundaplasty must be expected to be less effective, and the cure of preexistent gangrenous lesions will be questionable. The more distally the collaterals enter the main artery, the less effective is the profundaplasty, even when PA and lower leg arteries are free from arteriosclerotic disease (Gautier and Bonneton 1971; Boren et al. 1980; Towne et al. 1981; Rollins et al. 1985). Consequently, when under these circumstances angiographic examination indicates that the distal PA or the lower leg arteries are suitable for anastomosis, a femoropopliteal or -crural bypass operation should be preferred.

The situation is more unfavorable, and the choice for either profundaplasty or distal bypass more difficult, if the quality of the distal PA and lower-leg arteries is poor as well. Under these circumstances, the choice of the procedure depends upon various factors, taking especially into account whether the quality of the distal PA and lower-leg arteries is good enough to perform a reliable anastomosis. (This can be demonstrated angiographically.)

The factors influencing the choice between profundaplasty and femorodistal bypass include:

1. General risk factors; age
2. Availability of autogenous (venous) reconstructive material
3. Access to operating area (primary or reoperation)
4. Quality of DFA
5. Quality of profundapopliteal collaterals and their entry sites
6. Suitability of distal PA or lower-leg arteries for anastomosis
7. Severity of limb ischemia

If (a) the general surgical risk is acceptable, (b) proper venous material is available for reconstruction, (c) the DFA and the DFA collaterals are of poor quality and the entry sites are affected by arteriosclerosis, (d) either the PA or any lower-leg arterial segment is of adequate quality for distal reconstruction, and (e) there are gangrenous lesions or pedal ischemic necrosis, a femoropopliteal or femorocrural bypass graft is the procedure of choice. In contrast, if (a) there are any serious general risk factors, (b) venous reconstructive material is lacking, (c) conditions for a distal bypass procedure are poor owing to impaired runoff or the bad condition of the lower-leg arteries, and (d) distal ischemic lesions are not too serious, a profundaplasty is preferable. Before a definite decision in favor of a profundaplasty is made, it is necessary to assess the outcome (see below).

Sometimes the goal of limb salvage will not be reached after profundaplasty and amputation is unavoidable. Then the profundaplasty can still prove to have been beneficial, because it may contribute – even under very unfavorable circumstances – to shift the level of amputation to a more distal part of the limb. In some cases, lowering the level of amputation from above the knee to below it is an indication to perform a profundaplasty.

Prediction of Success After Profundaplasty

Sufficient improvement in distal limb perfusion to reduce intermittent claudication, significantly relieve rest pain, and/or permit healing of ischemic ulcers or healing of gangrenous areas primarily or after debridement or minor amputations must be achieved to justify selection of produndaplasty rather than femoropopliteal or -crural bypass. Several criteria relate to the success of isolated profundaplasty and should be evaluated carefully both preoperatively and at surgery in order to select operative candidates properly.

Iliac arterial and CFA inflow must be unimpaired as established by the quality of the femoral pulse, angiography, or duplex scanning and determination of the aortofemoral pressure gradient.

A well-developed profundapopliteal collateral bed and unimpaired popliteotibial runoff vessels are other important prerequisites for success.

It is possible to assess the presence and quantity of the profundapopliteal collaterals by angiography. The quality and hemodynamic value of the profundapopliteal collateral system can be determined by functional tests.

Bernhard et al. (1976) and Baron et al. (1981) recommended intraoperative measurements of DFA blood flow after intra-arterial injection of papaverine hydrochloride. They claim that this test is a practical and accurate procedure not only for evaluating the success of the profundaplasty, but also for obtaining information concerning the inflow tract of the vessel being reconstructed and the quality of blood supply ("blood flow potential of the DFA").

Preoperatively, the capacity of the profundapopliteal collateral system can be determined by noninvasive segmental pressure measurements (Boren et al. 1980; Rollins et al. 1985). The systolic pressure is measured above and below the knee and the profundapopliteal collateral index (PPCI) is calculated from these pressures by using the formula

$$\mathrm{PPCI} = \frac{\text{AK pressure} - \text{BK pressure}}{\text{AK pressure}}$$

This index reflects the resistance of the collateral bed. A high index, more than 0.5, due to a high pressure gradient across the knee, suggests poor collateral development and predicts poor success of profundaplasty to salvage a severely ischemic foot. A low index, less than 0.25, indicates a reasonable chance for a good result.

The patency and quality of the popliteotibial runoff can be demonstrated by arteriography. An unimpaired popliteotibial runoff usually correlates with success, whereas extensive occlusive disease of the runoff arteries is frequently associated with failure.

The importance of adequate arteriographic examination should not be underestimated. Arteriography allows the patency and quality of the inflow vessels to be judged as well as the PA with its collateral recipient segment, the lower-leg arteries, and the DFA itself. Moreover, arteriography provides an impression of the quantity of profundapopliteal collaterals. In this connection it must be emphasized that arteriographic assessment also has a prognostic value. It reliably predicts a successful profundaplasty when the following conditions exist: (a) an unimpaired iliac arterial and CFA inflow tract, (b) significant stenosis of the proximal DFA, (c) minimal arteriosclerotic lesions of the distal DFA, (d) a well-developed profundapopliteal collateral system, (e) patent PA and unimpaired popliteal recipient segment, and (f) minimal crural outflow occlusive disease.

All clinical, arteriographic, and hemodynamic criteria contribute to the identification of those patients in whom profundaplasty will be most effective and to the determination of the long-term durability of profundaplasty performed to effect limb salvage.

Old and New Operative Procedures

There are many methods of profundaplasty (Dos Santos 1966; Martin et al. 1968; van Dongen and Schwilden 1974; Schwilden and van Dongen 1989; van Dongen 1990). The simplest is antegrade removal of the sclerotic thickening and plaques from the proximal portion of the DFA through an arteriotomy in the CFA (Fig. 5).

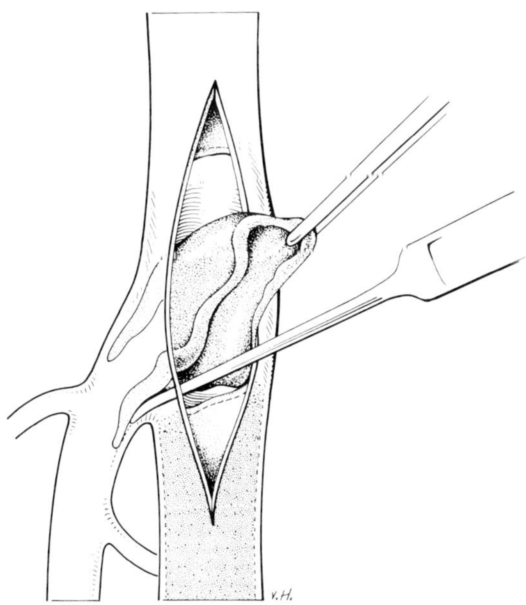

Fig. 5. Antegrade removal of the thickened intima and plaques from the proximal portion of the deep femoral artery (DFA) ("transfemoral unplugging")

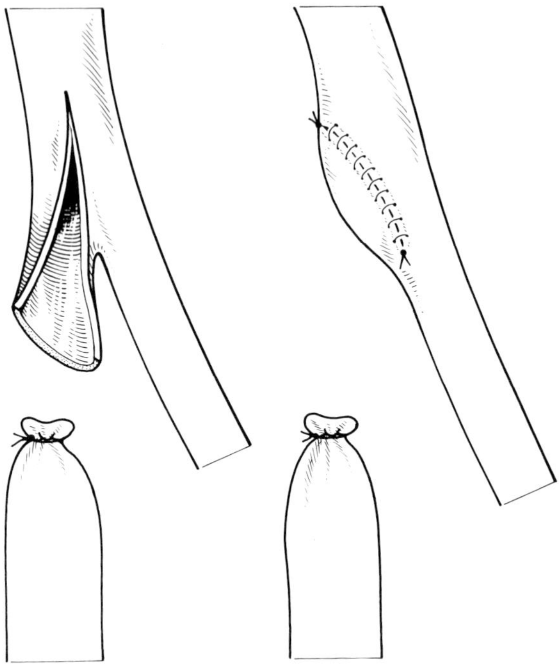

Fig. 6. Use of a pedicled flap of the wall of the endarterectomized superficial femoral artery (SFA) reflected upward, as proposed by Denck in 1966

However, the results of this so-called transfemoral unplugging (Morris et al. 1961; Martin et al. 1972; Thompson et al. 1977) are poor. Moreover, patency of the artery is endangered by a loose distal intimal edge, remnants of plaques, fragments of pathologic intima, and tabs of the media. All these remnants and irregularities can be the cause of thrombotic occlusion. Antegrade disobliteration of the DFA is inadequate, dangerous, and consequently inacceptable.

Denck (1966) was one of the first vascular surgeons to describe a real profundaplasty. He used a pedicled flap of the wall of the endarterectomized SFA reflected upward and sutured into the CFA wall (Fig. 6). Using this procedure, however, none of the morphologic or hemodynamic hindrances to flow are eliminated. Factors causing turbulence become even more important, because the difference in caliber between the CFA and DFA increases.

In 1966, Waibel introduced three different profundaplasties. The first also makes use of a pedicled flap of the wall of the endarterectomized proximal SFA, but this flap is sutured into the wall of the proximal DFA (Fig. 7). The lumen of the DFA can

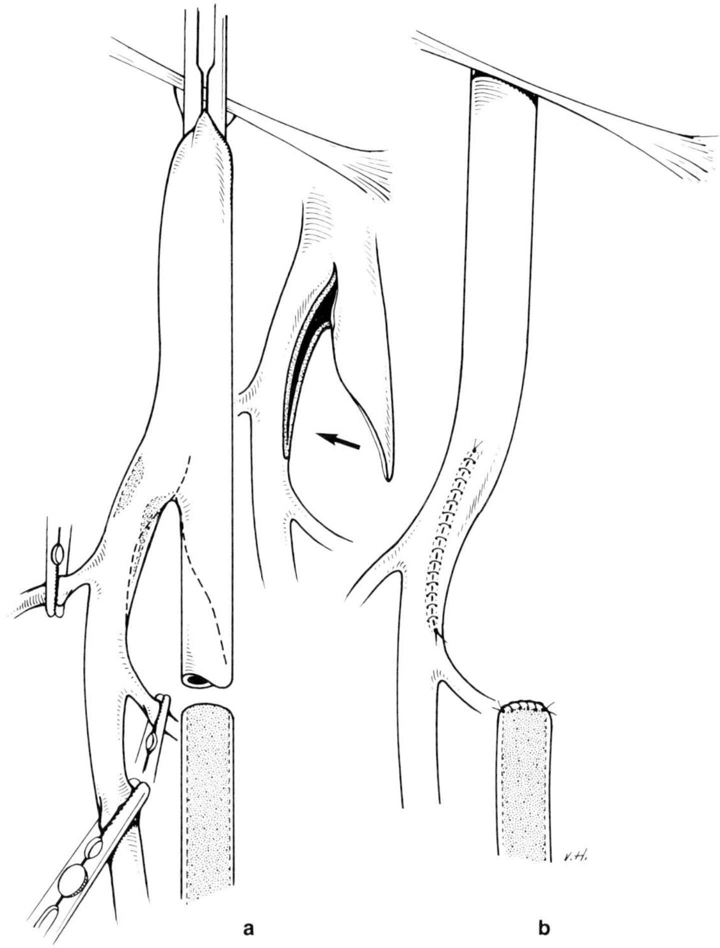

Fig. 7a,b. Pedicled flap of the wall of the endarterectomized proximal superficial femoral artery (SFA) sutured into the wall of the proximal deep femoral artery (DFA) as described by Waibel in 1966 ("beak patch profundaplasty")

be sufficiently enlarged by this autogenous arterial flap graft procedure, which is called "beak patch profundaplasty."

The second method described by Waibel is an autogenous SFA in situ bypass construction in which the proximal portion of the DFA is bridged with an endarterectomized part of the proximal SFA (Fig. 8).

In the third profundaplasty suggested by Waibel, enlargement of the proximal DFA is achieved by distal displacement of the femoral bifurcation. The walls of the proximal DFA and SFA facing each other are incised over a short distance as far as beyond

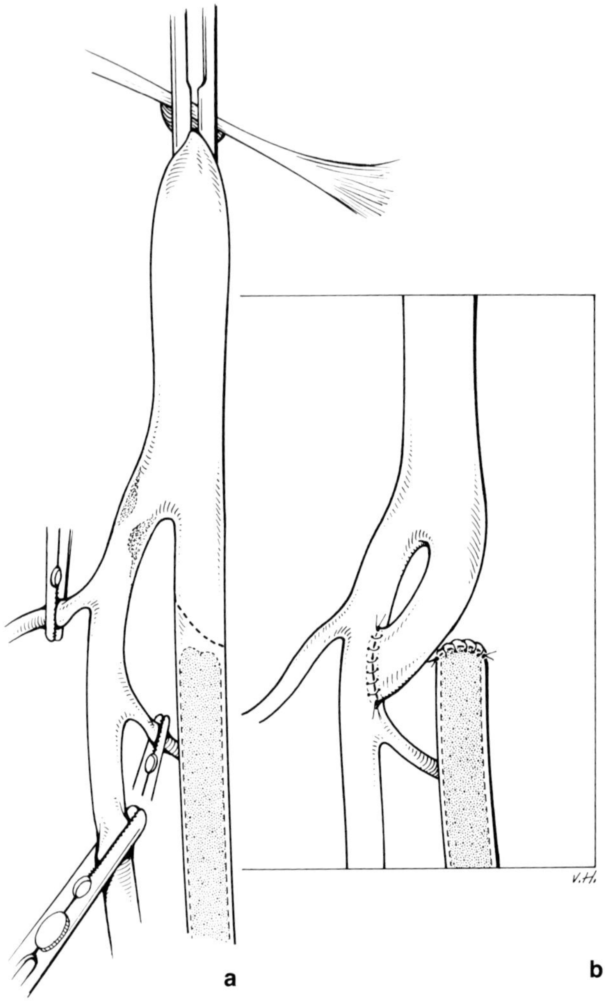

Fig. 8a,b. The narrowed portion of the deep femoral artery (DFA) is bridged with an endarterectomized portion of the proximal superficial femoral artery (SFA) ("autogenous SFA in situ bypass construction" as proposed by Waibel in 1966)

the stenotic area. At the back wall the edges are sutured together and at the front a vein patch is sutured in (Fig. 9). It is a technically difficult and time-consuming procedure.

Using all these techniques it is possible to eliminate the pathologic arteriosclerotic stenosis in the proximal DFA and the kinking of the blood at the origin of the DFA, but all other obstacles remain unchanged, especially the sources of turbulence and the geometric stenosis. In many cases turbulence even increases.

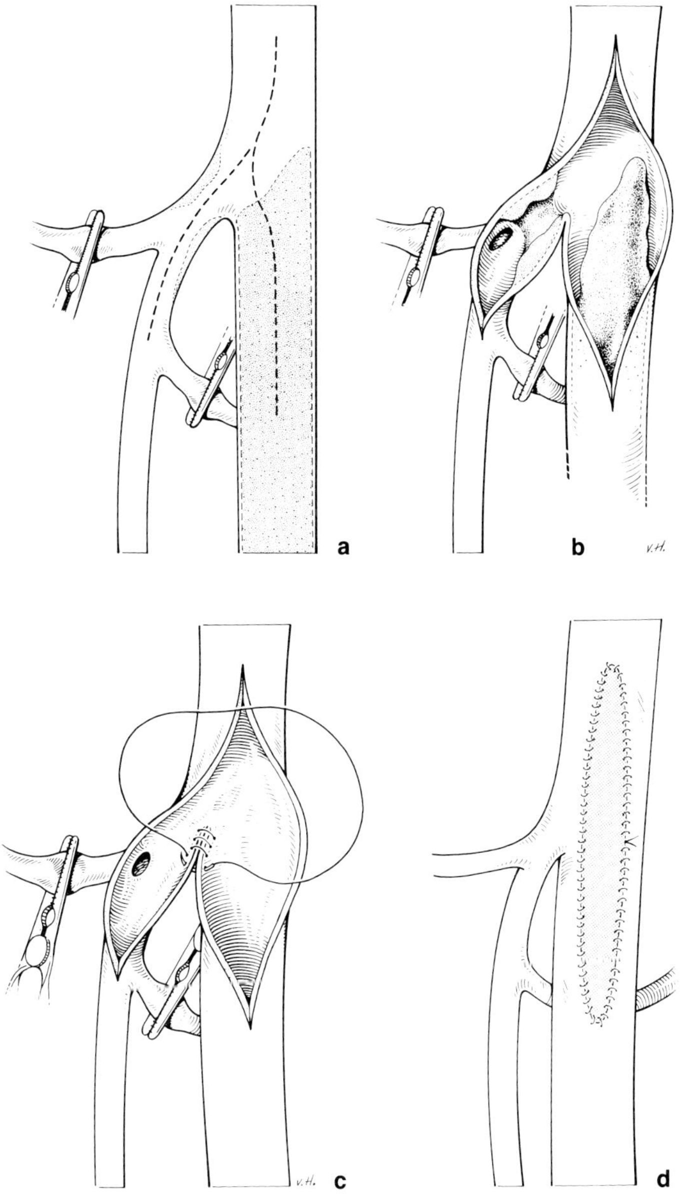

Fig. 9a–d. Enlargement of the proximal deep femoral artery (DFA) by distally displacement of the femoral bifurcation (Waibel 1966). **a** Y-shaped incision. **b** Opening of the femoral bifurcation. **c** Back wall suture. **d** Insertion of venous patch graft at the front

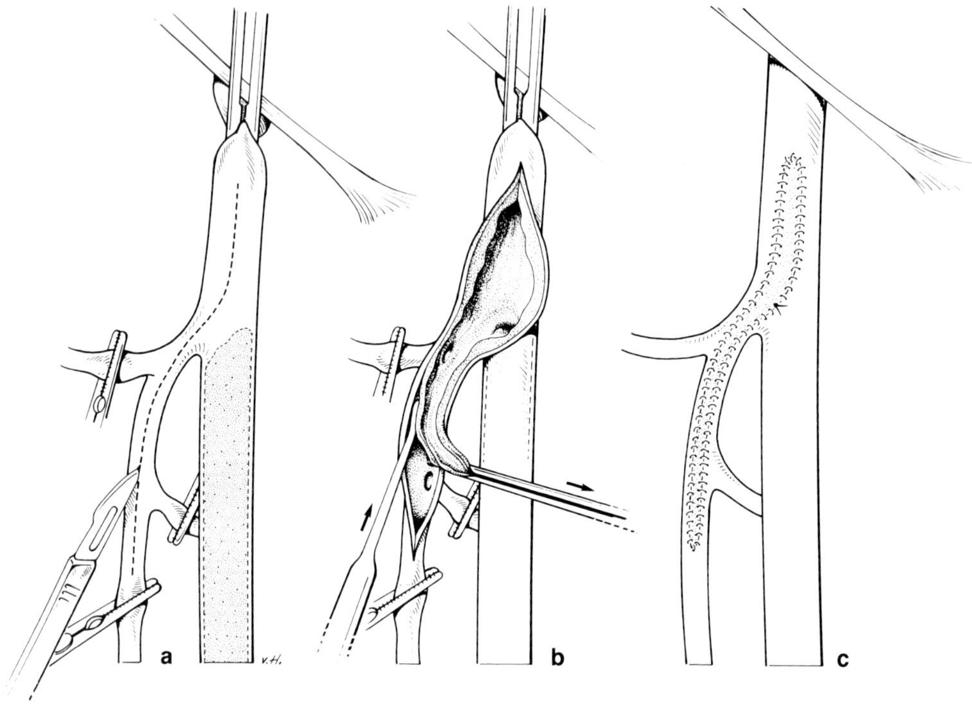

Fig. 10a–c. Technique of the patch graft profundaplasty ("hockey stick patch," "banana patch," or "boomerang patch" profundaplasty) proposed by Martin in 1968

More simple is the patch graft profundaplasty propagated by Martin and coworkers (Martin et al. 1968; Martin 1972). After an incision has been made from the CFA into the wall of the DFA at the level of the arteriosclerotic stenosis, a local open endarterectomy is performed, after which the lumen is enlarged by suturing in a venous patch ("hockey stick patch," "banana patch," or "boomerang patch" profundaplasty) (Fig. 10). This method is still used by many vascular surgeons, but the results are disappointing. This is not surprising, because only the organic arteriosclerotic narrowing is eliminated by this procedure. All other causes of impeded flow remain unchanged.

A hemodynamic weak point of the boomerang patch graft and other profundaplasties is the origin of the SFA. The hemodynamically unfavorable, sharply bending dorsolateral takeoff of the DFA remains unchanged. The kink in the conduit can be eliminated somewhat by dividing the SFA in its proximal portion (Fig. 11). However, the stump of the SFA with the thrombus is

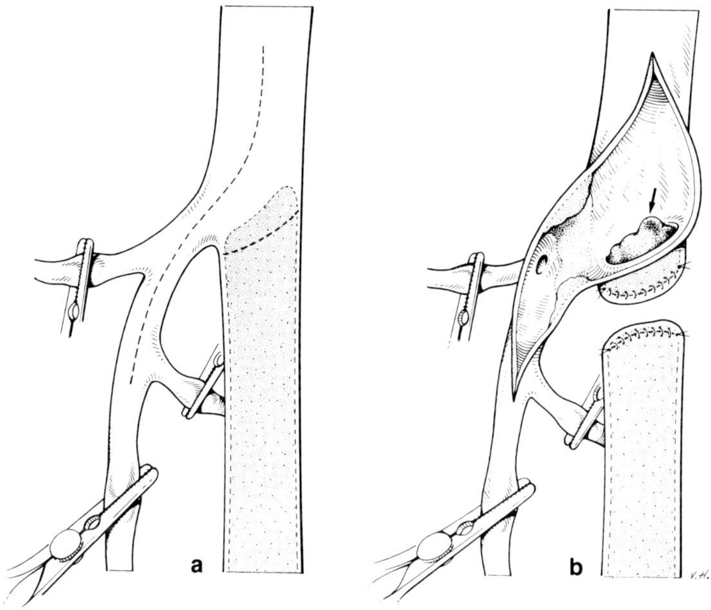

Fig. 11a,b. Transection of the first portion of the superficial femoral artery (SFA) and oversewing of the proximal stump so as to eliminate the kink in the conduit

left behind and this stump is still a source of turbulence and thrombosis. If this stump is endarterectomized, the result is a dead space, which causes turbulence or thrombosis with possible progression into the lumen of the CFA bifurcation. Attempts have been made to prevent these complications by proximal transection of the SFA at its origin and suture of the remaining stump (Fig. 12). By doing so, the turbulent flow at the transition of the CFA into the DFA can be transformed into a laminar flow. However, a disadvantage is that suture of the friable edges of the SFA origin is frequently the cause of hemorrhage and false aneurysm formation. For this reason this method was soon rejected.

van Dongen and Schwilden (1974) solved this problem by excising the origin of the SFA from the DFA arteriotomy (Fig. 13). They called this the resectional profundaplasty. This procedure differs from the usual boomerang patch graft profundaplasty inasmuch as local problems occurring at the femoral bifurcation, e.g., dorsolateral kinking, intimal dissection, or local thrombosis, are eliminated by excising the origin of the SFA. This maneuver creates superior hemodynamic conditions.

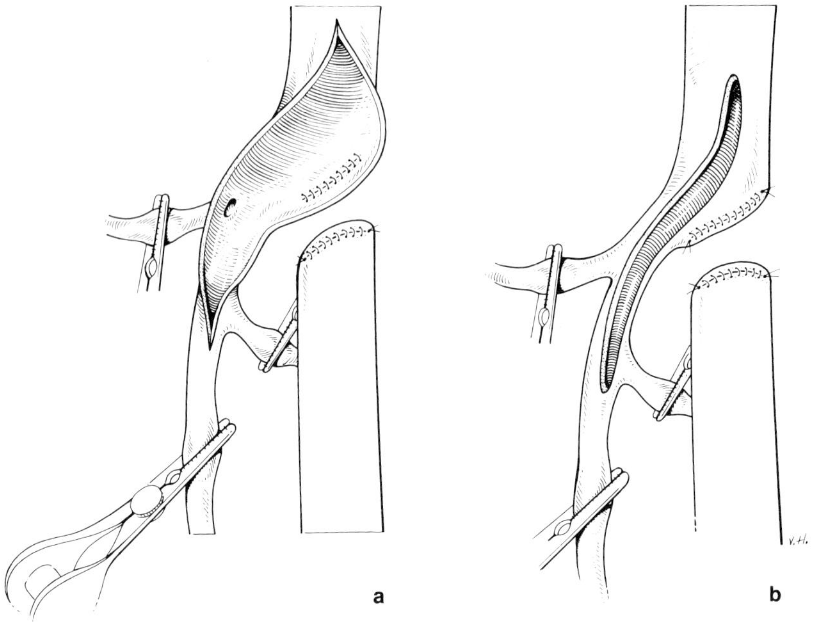

Fig. 12a,b. Excision of the origin of the superficial femoral artery (SFA) from the wall of the femoral bifurcation and closure of the opening with the intention of eliminating a source of turbulence and thrombosis

Operative Technique of the Extended Resectional Profundaplasty

Positioning

Operations on the DFA are done with the patient in supine position with abduction and slight external rotation of the thigh and the knee slightly flexed. The exposition of the groin region is reinforced by placing a soft pillow under the pelvis at the opposite side and a second pillow under the knee (Fig. 13a). This relaxes the muscles overlying the DFA. To prevent ischemic decubital necrosis during the operation, the feet should be wrapped in cotton dressing. When draping, one must always consider vein harvesting. Venous material for patch grafts should under no circumstances be taken from the inguinal portion of the great saphenous vein, but always from the region of the medial malleolus of the contralateral ankle. Harvesting from the ipsilateral leg may lead to impaired wound healing if ischemia is severe.

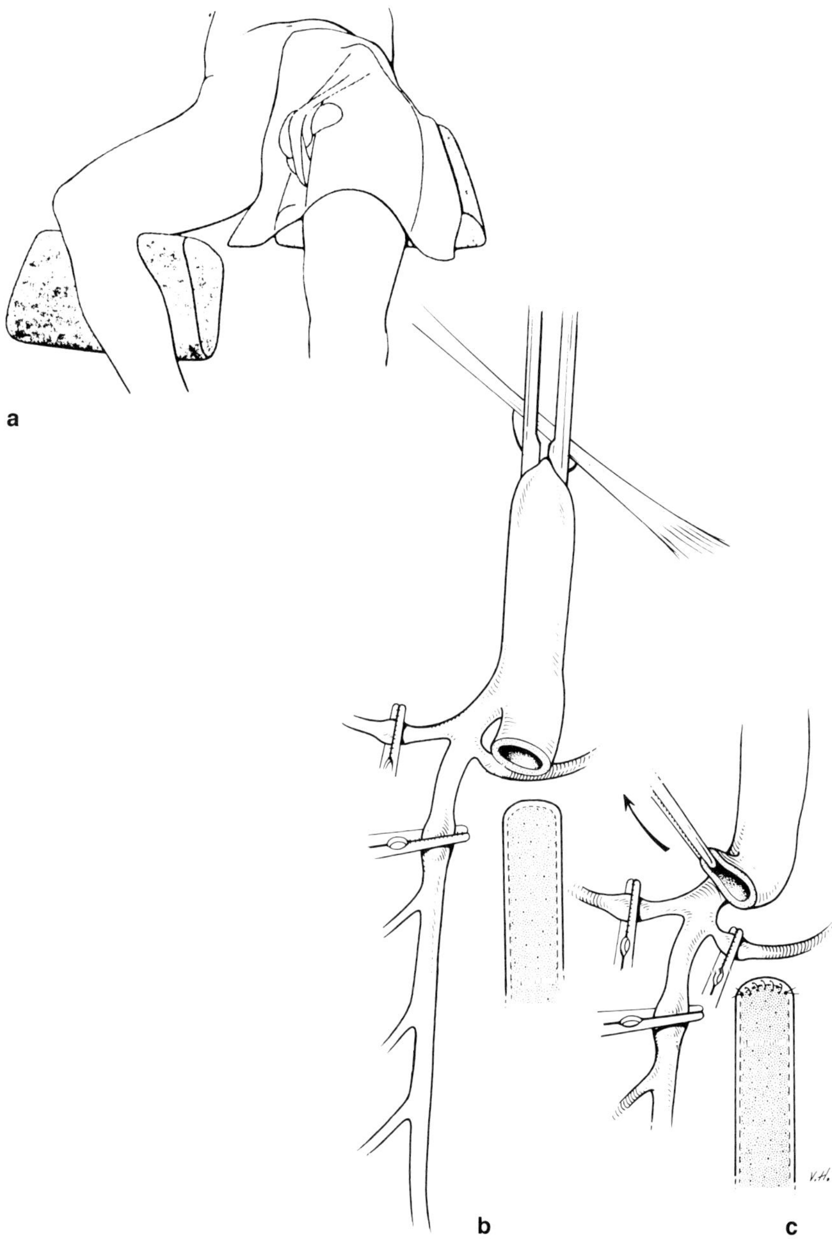

Fig. 13a–j. Technique of resectional profundaplasty. **a** Positioning of the patient. Abduction and slight external rotation of the thigh obtained by placing pillows under the knee joint and under the pelvis of the opposite side. **b** Transection of the occluded superficial femoral artery (SFA) about 1 cm distal to its origin. Identification and clamping of the lateral circumflex artery. **c** The proximal stump of the SFA is rotated anteriorly. Identification and clamping of the medial femoral circumflex artery

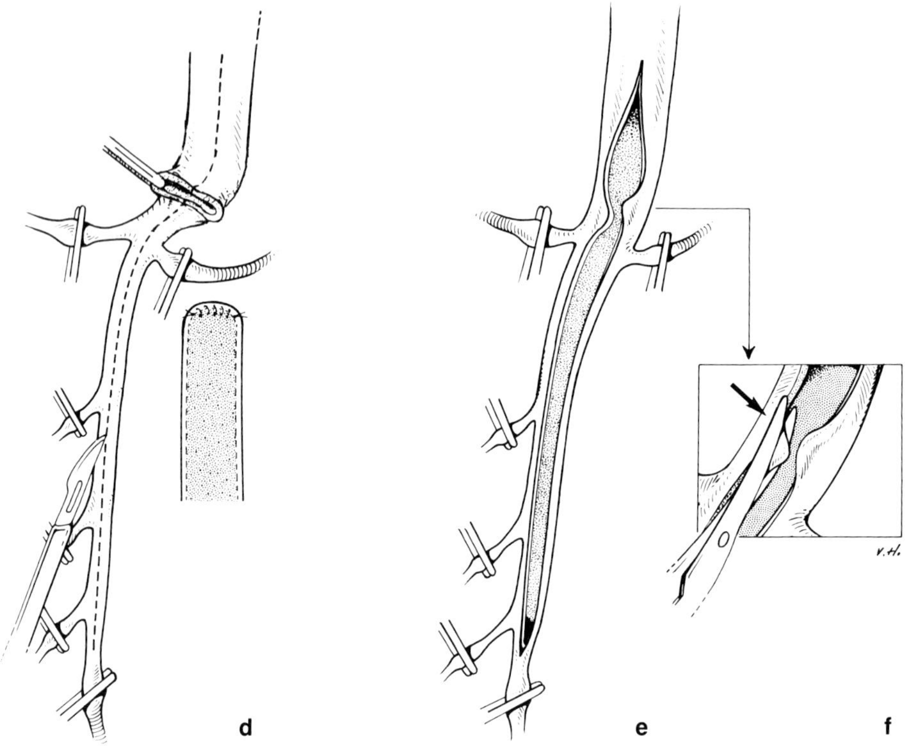

Fig. 13 *Continued* **d,e** Incision of the anterior wall of the deep femoral artery (DFA) at least 3 cm distal to the bifurcation and extension of the incision proximally through the origin of the SFA up to the clamp beneath the inguinal ligament and distally beyond the last geometrically relevant branch of the DFA, preferably the last perforating branch. **f** Removal of the remnants of the origin of the SFA on either side (as limited as possible)

Approach to the Deep Femoral Artery

A standard longitudinal skin incision is made over the CFA. Distally the incision is extended across the sartorius muscle (Hershey and Auer 1974; Rollins et al. 1985; Schwilden and van Dongen 1989). Dissection of the CFA and SFA is carried out in the usual way. The origin of the DFA is identified and the tissue covering it is dissected. First, one or two thin venae comitantes crossing in front of the DFA are encountered and divided. Then, somewhat more distally, the lateral circumflex vein can be divided in front of the DFA. After division of this vein, the short stumps are ligated with transfixation ligatures. The first branches of the DFA, the lateral and medial femoral circumflex arteries, are exposed and

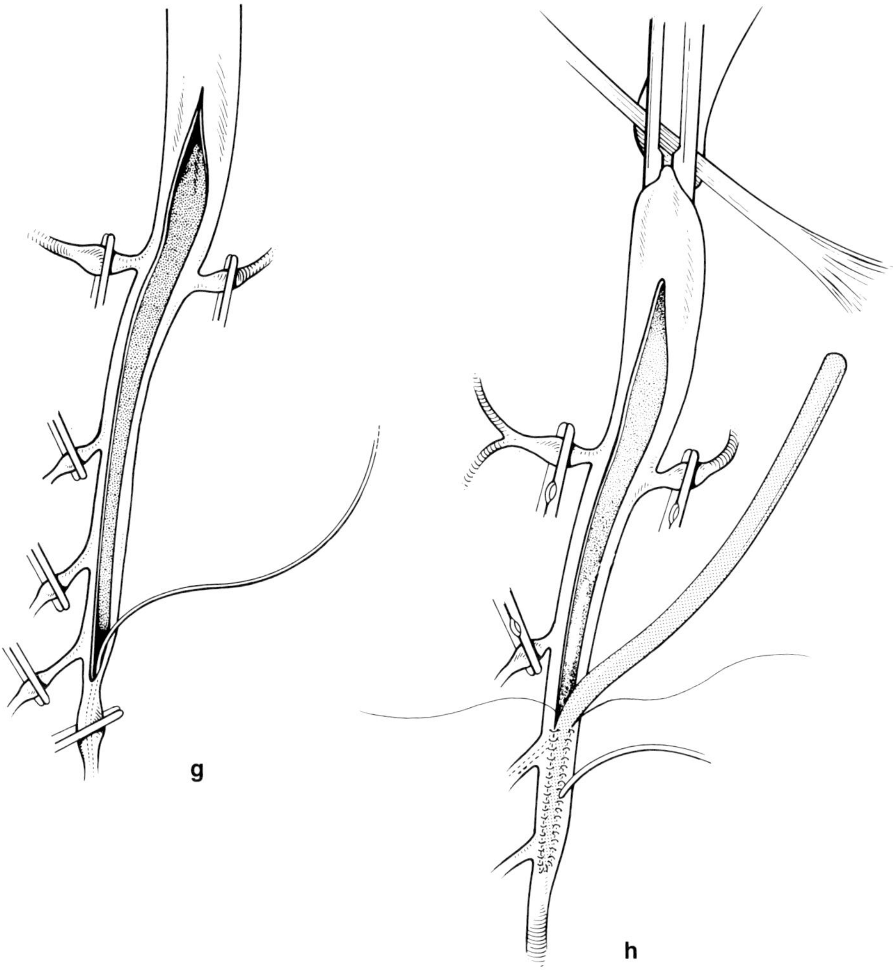

Fig. 13 *Continued* **g** The distal DFA is perfused with a heparinized saline solution through a thin catheter inserted distally between the jaws of a soft-closing bulldog clamp. **h** A venous patch is sutured into the wall opening starting at the distal corner of the arteriotomy

dissected carefully. They must be preserved, because they are important for collateral circulation.

Occasionally, with a low bifurcation of the CFA, the first and largest branch of the DFA, the medial or the lateral femoral circumflex artery, has a separate origin from the CFA (Vaas 1975). These variations are rarely troublesome.

The space between the femoral vessels on the medial side and the sartorius muscle on the lateral side is spread apart, and the DFA is dissected further distally in the deeper layers, carefully

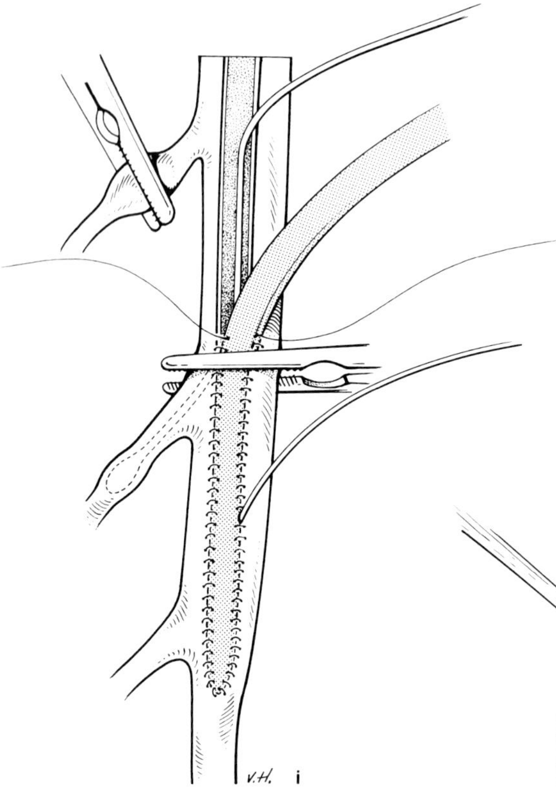

V.H. i

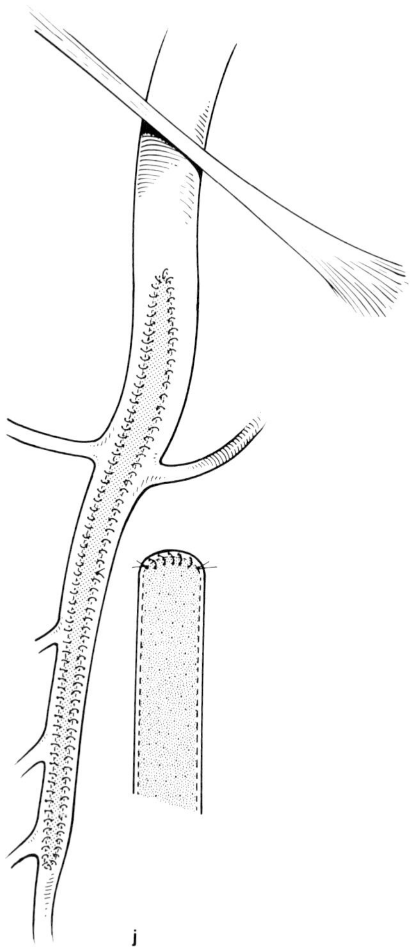

j

Fig. 13 *Continued* **i** The origin of all side branches are checked successively with a probe to be sure that they are open and functioning. **j** The profundaplasty completed and the clamp removed, it can be established that the common femoral artery (CFA) and the DFA are in a direct line, without kinking. The calibers of the CFA and DFA are adapted. All obstacles have been eliminated

avoiding damage to the muscular and cutaneous branches of the femoral nerve as well as the saphenous nerve. During dissection of the DFA, the deep femoral vein will be encountered crossing over the artery to empty into the superficial femoral vein. After division of its various muscular tributaries, it can be drawn aside with a small vein retractor to uncover the DFA more distally. While dissecting the DFA, all the perforating arteries are carefully identified and preserved. Every effort should be made to maintain the integrity of all branches, because the potential capacity of the profundapopliteal collateral system and consequently the success of the profundaplasty to be performed depends upon adequate flow through each of them. Finally, the DFA passes behind the adductor longus muscle. Usually the distally perforating artery originates from the trunk at this point, forming together with the continuation of the trunk the so-called distal bifurcation of the DFA. If necessary, the adductor longus muscle can be partially divided.

Resectional Profundaplasty

During the procedure, all branches of the DFA including the perforating arteries are occluded with extremely soft bulldog clamps that exert very gentle pressure on the vascular wall.

After 70 U heparin per kg bodyweight have been administrated intravenously, the proximal CFA is clamped with an atraumatic arterial clamp. The trunk of the DFA is prepared proximal to the origin of the first perforating branch, and the lateral femoral circumflex branch is occluded with soft bulldog clamps. The occluded SFA is transected about 1 cm distal to its origin (Fig. 13b). In the event of back bleeding, the distal stump is sutured atraumatically. The completely mobilized proximal stump of the SFA, branching off in a ventromedial direction, is gripped with forceps and rotated anteriorly (Fig. 13c). The medial femoral circumflex artery is identified in this way and is clamped with a soft bulldog clamp. Then the DFA is opened by a stab incision of the anterior wall at least 3 cm distal to the bifurcation (Fig. 13d). The incision is extended proximally through the origin of the SFA up the CFA until the proximal clamp beneath the inguinal ligament is reached. The remnants of the origin of the SFA are removed on either side in as limited a manner as possible (Fig. 13f). When the remnants are excised too much, the back wall of the DFA orifice will prove to be too narrow.

After clamping the second perforating artery and the branches of the distal bifurcation, the arteriotomy is extended distally beyond the geometrically relevant branch of the DFA, preferably the last perforating branch (Fig. 13e). To prevent clot formation due to blood stasis, the distal DFA trunk is perfused with heparinized saline solution through a thin catheter (Fig. 13g).

Starting in the proximal DFA, the atheromatously thickened intima is loosened in the cleavage plain using a sharp dissector. The dissection is continued proximally halfway up the CFA. There the thickened intima is tapered off as flatly and smoothly as possible using a sharp scalpel. The diseased intima is carefully dissected from the "threshold" at the transition of the CFA into the DFA.

The distal dissection occurs mostly by itself when the disobliterated intima is lifted, because the thickened intima gradually changes into the normal distal intimal layer. During the dissection, most branches of the DFA will be opened. When the intimal thickening proceeds into a branch or if the orifices of the branches are also narrowed by arteriosclerotic debris, everything should be done to normalize blood flow through these orifices. Normally, antegrade removal of the sclerotic lesion, which usually extends only a few millimeters into the branches, is facilitated by careful eversion of the side branches into the lumen of the DFA.

If the intima of the mid- and distal portion of the DFA trunk is only slightly thickened, relatively smooth, not ulcerated, and not irregular, it should not be removed totally. In such cases the endarterectomy can be restricted to the proximal portion of the DFA. At the distal end of the endarterectomy, the intima is cut obliquely and flat with a sharp scalpel at the most suitable point, just proximal to the take off of a side branch. There, the distal intimal edge is by nature firmly fixed to the vessel wall around the orifice of the branch and cannot be loosened by the force of the blood stream. The advantage of this confined intimectomy is that most of the intima – the best protection of the inner surface – is preserved, which is important especially in the narrow distal half of the DFA.

Following the endarterectomy a venous patch, harvested from the greater saphenous vein at the level of the medial malleolus of the opposite limb, is prepared, slightly dilated with heparinized blood, cut along its full length, and trimmed to the appropriate width: 4–5 mm. The patch graft should be appropriately tailored, narrowing distally. A patch which is too wide may lead to formation of a false aneurysm. Prosthetic material should never be used as patch graft in the wall of the DFA. If no greater saphenous vein is available, a segment of the short saphenous vein or the cephalic vein is a useful alternative. If required, an arterial patch can be tailored from a resected and endarterectomized segment of the obstructed proximal SFA.

Starting at the distal angle of the arteriotomy, the venous patch is sutured in (Fig. 13h). First, the bluntly rounded end of the patch is fixed at the most critical point, the distal corner of the arteriotomy, using two or three interrupted sutures. Then the patch is fixed by continuous over and over sutures on either side; 7–0 suture material is used.

If braided material is chosen, the stitch direction should be from the artery to the vein. When the venous patch is perforated first from the outside to the inside, thrombogenic adventitial fibers may be dragged by the braided suture into the stitch holes and get on the luminal side of the patch. Under unfavorable circumstances (reduced blood flow) this may induce thrombosis. When using monofilament smooth suture material, dragging of adventitial tissue into the lumen does not occur. During the time needed for suturing in a patch graft, the perfusion of the distal DFA with heparinized saline solution should be continued.

When about 5 cm of the vein patch graft has been sutured in, the patched part of the artery is flushed with heparin saline solution to remove blood clots. A new bulldog clamp is then placed on the patched trunk just distal to the last stitches on either side, and the clamps occluding the distal branches are removed, allowing the finished part of the angioplasty to fill with (heparinized) blood (Fig. 13i). With a probe introduced into the lumen of the patched part of the angioplasty (Fig. 13i), the patency of the origins of all side branches is checked to be sure that these important runoff vessels are functioning well.

Then the patch graft is sutured in further proximally, again over a distance of about 5 cm, after which the bulldog clamps are moved proximally. In this way the vein patch is sutured in part by part, until the proximal corner of the arteriotomy has been reached. When the sutures are completed, blood flow through the DFA is restored by removing all clamps (Fig. 13j).

Once the profundaplasty has been completed it can be seen that the situation has changed strikingly (Fig. 14). The CFA and DFA are in a straight line. A gradual conical transition of the CFA into the DFA is created, without kinking of the conduit at the site of the former takeoff of the DFA. The calibers of the CFA and DFA are adapted; there is no abrupt reduction of diameter between the CFA and DFA. The DFA is enlarged over its entire length,

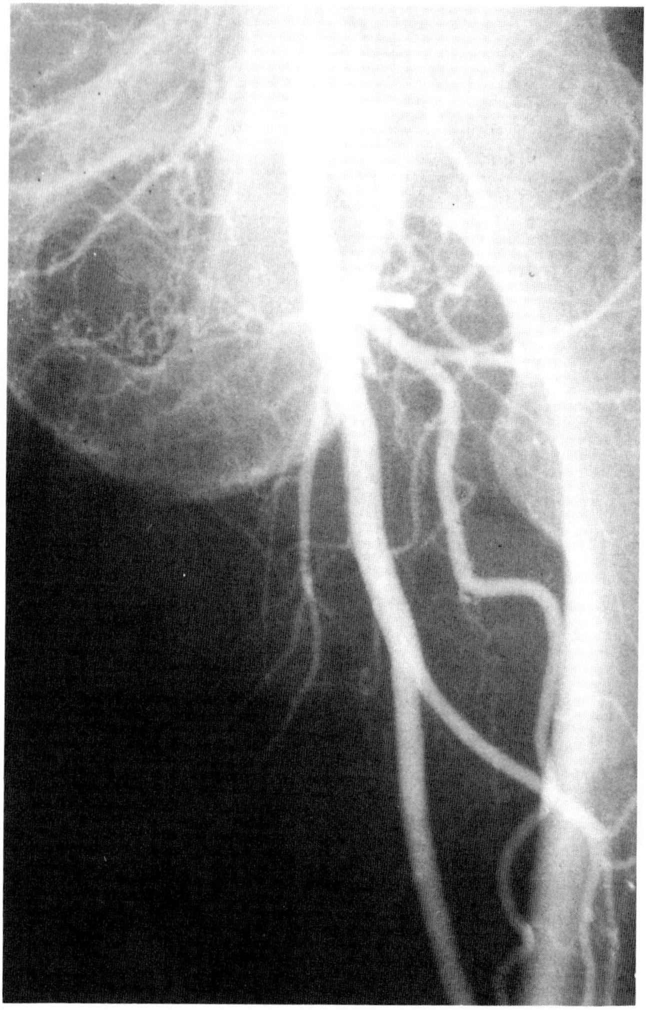

Fig. 14. Arteriographic appearance of the common femoral artery (CFA) and the deep femoral artery (DFA) after extended resectional profundaplasty

but the gradual reduction of lumen in distal direction is maintained. Hemodynamics are surprisingly good. All sources of turbulence are eliminated. The turbulent flow has changed into a undisturbed laminar one, as was demonstrated by Maurer and coworkers (1979). All hemodynamic, pathological, geometric, and anatomical obstacles are eliminated.

Additional Measures

Following the profundaplasty a lumbar sympathectomy may be carried out, although the value of this combination is not based on data from prospective clinical studies. It is our opinion that the dubious beneficial effect of an additional sympathectomy does not merit the increased postoperative morbidity. Profundaplasty is a simple and minor procedure requiring only a short operation time and should not be enhanced by a more burdening operative intervention.

Anticoagulant and/or antiplatelet therapy is recommended in all patients. The value of long-term oral anticoagulants is not supported by reliable clinical evidence. Nevertheless, some authors attach value to it.

Antibiotics are employed in the presence of infected lesions of the foot. Specific antibiotics are administered as determined by results of preoperative culture and sensitivity tests. The appropriate drugs are started prior to surgery, and they are continued throughout the operation and for at least 7 days postoperatively.

Results

From 1975 to 1987, 452 patients underwent isolated profundaplasties. Three hundred and eighty-six patients had a unilateral profundaplasty, and in 66 patients a bilateral operation was performed. Altogether, profundaplasties were carried out in 518 limbs. Four hundred and seventy-two limbs (91%) underwent a primary profundaplasty. A secondary profundaplasty was performed in 46 limbs (9%), in most cases after failure of a femoropopliteal or -crural bypass operation. Mean age of the patients was 63 years, with a range of 50–88 years. The group consisted of 372 men (82%) and 80 women (18%). One hundred and ten (24.6%) were diabetic.

After deduction of early postoperative mortality (five deaths representing six limbs), 447 patients (512 limbs) were available for follow-up studies (Table 2). In 62% of limbs the indication for surgery was disabling intermittent claudication, in 16% rest pain, and in 22% ischemic ulcers, gangrenous lesions, or pedal ischemic necrosis.

An excisional profundaplasty was performed in 407 limbs (Table 2). For the purpose of analysis, the length of the profund-

Table 2. Methods of profundaplasty performed in 512 limbs of 447 surviving patients, related to severity of symptoms

Method of profundaplasty	Limbs (*n*)	Severity of ischemic symptoms		
		Intermittent claudication	Rest pain	Ischemic ulcers, gangrenous lesions
Profundaplasty with resection of the origin of the SFA	407			
Short	110	92	13	5
Partially extended	109	72	14	23
Extended	188	78	36	74
Boomerang patch profundaplasty	68	50	9	9
Beak patch profundaplasty	15	8	6	1
Other profundaplasties	22	16	4	2
Total of limbs	512 (100%)	316 (62%)	82 (16%)	114 (22%)

SFA, superficial femoral artery.

aplasty was divided into short (beyond the lateral circumflex branch), partially extended (beyond the first or second perforating artery), and extended (until the last perforating artery). A short resectional profundaplasty was carried out in 110 legs, a partially extended one in 109, and an extended profundaplasty in 188 limbs. Generally considered, the extent of the profundaplasty correlates with the severity of ischemic symptoms (Table 2). In all cases the SFA was occluded or seriously narrowed. A boomerang patch graft profundaplasty was performed in 68 limbs – legs with an extremely stenotic, but still functioning SFA. In these cases it is not justifiable to sacrifice this artery, so a resectional profundaplasty could not be considered. In 15 limbs, a beak patch graft profundaplasty was performed. Other profundaplasties were used in 22 limbs. Preoperative studies included aortobifemoral angiography, ankle–brachial pressure index measurements, and measurement of walking ability on the treadmill. Preoperative PPCI values were available in 231 patients. Basal and papaverine-augmented blood flows were measured intraoperatively before and after profundaplasty in all limbs. Adequacy of inflow was assessed preoperatively by palpation of femoral pulses, review of arteriograms, and in many cases pressure and flow measurements. All patients were treated postoperatively with anticoagulants (coumarine), in principle until death, unless anticoagulation was contraindicated. The patients were followed until 31 December 1989, or until death, with clinical and vascular laboratory studies. The minimum observation time was 2 years.

Mortality, Complications, and Patency Rate

Operative and early postoperative mortality for all profundaplasties was 1.1% (five patients representing six limbs) (Table 3). Deaths were confined to those patients in desperate need of operation to prevent major operations. There were no deaths among patients operated on for claudication. All deaths were in the limb salvage group. Three deaths were due to myocardial infarction, one (with bilateral profundaplasty) to pulmonary embolism, and one to pulmonary insufficiency. The low mortality rate may be due to the relatively short operating time required, the technical simplicity of the procedure, and the slight burden for the patient. Moreover, the procedure can be carried out with epidural or local anesthesia combined with superficial general anesthesia.

Postoperative complications were noted in 36 of the 447 surviving patients (8.1%; Table 3). Early thrombosis occurred in eight patients (1.8%), and thrombectomy or thrombolysis was performed successfully in seven of them. In one case this treatment was unsuccessful, but the patient in question obviously had sufficient collateral circulation, so that the limb could be salvaged. Hemorrhage occurred in seven patients (1.6%). In all cases operative revision and correction was successful, but was followed by wound infection in three patients.

A profundaplasty can be considered patent if the femoral pulse is fully palpable and if there is an increase in the ankle–brachial index of at least 0.2. The DFA is considered to be occluded if the femoral pulse has disappeared or if the ankle–brachial index has

Table 3. Mortality and early postoperative complications in 452 patients treated with profundaplasty

Complication	Patients	
	(*n*)	(%)
Mortality	5	1.1
Myocardial infarction	6	1.4
Pulmonary insufficiency	5	1.1
Thrombosis of angioplasty	8	1.8
Hemorrhage	7	1.6
Wound infection	10	2.3
Infection of angioplasty	0	0.0
Total	36	8.1

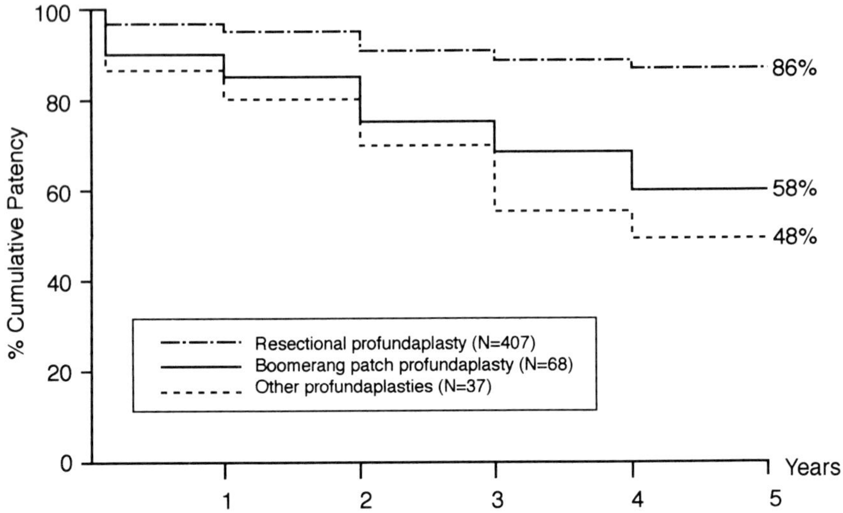

Fig. 15. Life-table patency rates for 407 resectional profundaplasties, 68 boomerang patch profundaplasties, and 37 other profundaplasties

returned to preoperative levels. Failure can be demonstrated by intravenous digital subtraction angiography.

Cumulative patency of the resectional profundaplasties was 97.0% at 30 days, but decreased to 85.8% at 5 years (Fig. 15). Cumulative patency rates of the boomerang patch and other profundaplasties were lower. The better patency rates of the resectional profundaplasties must be attributed to the more favorable hemodynamic conditions and the higher flow rates of the resectional procedures. Higher flow rates are presumed favorable for long-term patency.

Vascular Laboratory Studies

Exercise testing has a restricted value in appreciating the functional disability due to arterial obstruction. The walking distance on the treadmill (set at 3.2 km/h, with a 7% slope) was measured to the onset of claudication pain in 268 patients with intermittent claudication before and after successful isolated profundaplasty. The average walking distance of these patients before surgery was 53 m (range, 5–120 m). Table 4 shows the mean walking times 6–12 weeks after the different methods of profundaplasty. Best

Table 4. Pre- and postoperative mean walking distances (meters) in 268 patients operated on for intermittent claudication

Kind of profundaplasty	Limbs (n)	Preoperative walking distance (m)		Postoperative walking distance (m)		Increase (%)
		Mean	Range	Mean	Range	
Resectional						
Short	68	65	10–110	200	120–>1000	208
Partially extended	65	50	10–95	225	80–>1000	350
Extended	70	45	5–100	300	85–>1000	567
Boomerang patch graft	45	60	10–120	170	80–>1000	183
Others	20	55	15–90	160	75–240	190

results were obtained after resectional profundaplasty, especially after the extended procedure.

Intraoperative flow rate measurements were performed in all patients (518 limbs) before and after the different methods of profundaplasty. Baseline as well as papaverine-augmented blood flows were measured.

Figure 16 shows the postreconstruction baseline as well as the postreconstruction papaverine-augmented blood flows after the different variants of profundaplasty as compared with the prereconstruction flow rates. After extended resectional profundaplasty, the increase of baseline and papaverine-augmented blood flow is highest, much higher than after short resectional and other profundaplasties. After extended profundaplasty, baseline flow increases by more than 300% and papaverine-augmented flow by more than 400%. This means that the volume of flow through a DFA treated with extended excisional profundaplasty is equal to the flow which can be measured in a patent SFA, both before and after vasodilation produced by the intra-arterial administration of papaverine, and equal to twice the flow which can usually be measured through a femoropopliteal bypass.

Clinical Presentation

Profundaplasty, performed for relief of claudication, was judged to be a success if the patient reported more than 200% improvement of walking distance or complete relief of symptoms at the time of

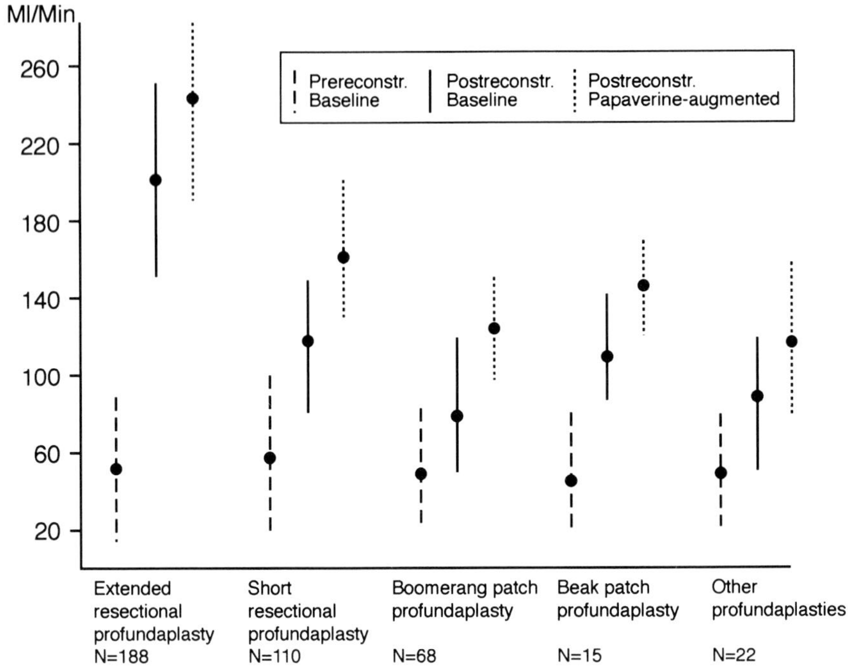

Fig. 16. Baseline and papaverine-augmented blood flows at the time of operation in 452 patients (518 limbs) before and after different methods of profundaplasty. Of the resectional profundaplasties, only blood flows of the short and extended angioplasties are shown. The values of the medium extended profundaplasties are between those of the short and extended procedures

follow-up control. Complete information was available for 268 out of 316 limbs operated upon for intermittent claudication (Tables 4 and 5).

Significant improvement or complete relief of claudication was achieved in 96% of the operated limbs, but improvement was more striking after the resectional profundaplasties, corresponding with the results of the exercise test on the treadmill. After resectional profundaplasty and especially after extended resectional profundaplasty, an unlimited walking distance (>1000 m) was obtained in 31% of limbs. Unlimited walking ability was reached in only 12 patients (4.5%) who underwent the other forms of profundaplasty. In most cases, it will be weeks or months before maximal improvement in walking distance or relief of claudication is achieved. The effect of profundaplasty will be more beneficial and will be noticeable sooner if after the operation a daily exercise and physical training program is started. In 11 patients (4.1%) no satisfactory improvement of severe claudication was obtained.

Table 5. Results of profundaplasty in patients operated on for claudication and rest pain

Indication	No. of patients	Success		Failure	
		(*n*)	(%)	(*n*)	(%)
Claudication	268	257	95.9	11	4.1
Rest pain	79	75	94.9	4	5.1

Table 6. Results of profundaplasty in 114 patients operated on for ischemic lesions and necrosis

Kind of profundaplasty	No. of patients	Ischemic ulcers			Ischemic necrosis		
		Limbs (*n*)	Healing		Limbs (*n*)	Healing	
			(*n*)	(%)		(*n*)	(%)
Resectional profundaplasty	102	47	40	85.1	55	41	74.5
– short	5	3	2	66.6	2	1	50.0
– partially extended	23	10	8	80.0	13	9	69.2
– extended	74	34	30	88.2	40	31	77.5
Other profundaplasties	12	4	1	25.0	8	2	25.0
Total	114	51	41	80.4	63	43	68.3

Eight of these patients underwent a distal bypass operation. There were no amputations in this group of patients.

Seventy five (94.9%) out of 79 patients operated upon for rest pain were rid of it after profundaplasty (Table 5). At 3 years the relief of rest pain was maintained in 86% of the patients after resectional profundaplasty, compared to 52% of the group of patients treated with other profundaplasties.

Profundaplasty in patients with ischemic defects of the foot were considered successful if the ischemic ulcers or the gangrenous or necrotic areas healed primarily or after debridement or minor amputation. Especially in these patients the superiority of the resectional profundaplasty (particularly of the extended one) was confirmed (Table 6). After extended profundaplasty, 88.2% of ischemic ulcers and 77.5% of ischemic necrotic and gangrenous lesions healed. Healing of these distal lesions was obtained in only a quarter of patients after performance of other nonresectional profundaplasties.

Table 7. Correlation of preoperative profundapopliteal collateral index (PPCI) values with results of profundaplasty in 193 limbs with rest pain or ischemic defects

Limb salvage	No. of limbs	Mean PPCI
Successful	159	0.18
Unsuccessful	34	0.48
Total	193	–

It must be emphasized that there was no significant difference between diabetic and nondiabetic patients.

Profundaplasty was not successful in achieving salvage in 34 out of 193 limbs with rest pain or ischemic defects (17.6%): four limbs with rest pain, ten with ischemic ulcers, and 20 with gangrenous or necrotic lesions. In these cases the possibility of a femorodistal bypass operation or the need for amputation must be considered. Twenty-four limbs did well after additional distal bypass procedure, but ten ultimately required amputation. Above-the-knee amputation was performed in only one patient. In all other patients, the amputation could be restricted to the lower leg (seven limbs) or the foot (two limbs), although in five of these limbs above-the-knee amputation was indicated as judged before profundaplasty. In these limbs profundaplasty had contributed to shifting the level of amputation to a more distal part of the limb.

The most important predictor of success or failure of profundaplasty for limb salvage was the PPCI. The PPCI was found to correlate well with the results of isolated profundaplasty when performed for limb salvage (Table 7). Successfully revascularized limbs had a mean PPCI of 0.18, compared with 0.48 in the limbs not salvaged by profundaplasty. The higher the PPCI, the more likely the operation was to fail.

References

Baron HC, Schwartz M, Batri G (1981) The papaverine test for blood flow potential of the profunda femoris artery. Surg Gynecol Obstet 153: 873–876

Beales JS, Adcock FA, Frawley JS et al (1971) The radiological assessment of disease of the profunda femoris artery. Br J Radiol 44: 854–859

Berguer R, Cotton LT, Higgins RF (1975a) Analysis of deep femoral artery hemodynamics and the affect of reconstruction. J Cardiovasc Surg 16: 148–149

Berguer R, Higgins RF, Cotton LT (1975b) Geometry, blood flow, and reconstruction of the deep femoral artery. Am J Surg 130: 68–73

Bernhard VM, Ray LI, Militello JP (1976) The role of angioplasty of the profunda femoris artery in revascularization of the ischemic limb. Surg Gynecol Obstet 142: 840–844

Boren CH, Towne JB, Bernhard VM, Salles-Cunha S (1980) Profundapopliteal collateral index. A guide to successful profundaplasty. Arch Surg 115: 1366–1371

David TE, Drezner AD (1978) Extended profundaplasty for limb salvage. Surgery 84: 758–762

Denck H (1966) Verbesserung der Durchblutung der unteren Extremität durch Profundaplastik. Acta Chir 1: 293–298

Dos Santos JC (1966) A critical review on the round table on endarterectomy. J Cardiovasc Surg 7: 307–321

Gautier R, Bonneton G (1971) La chirurgie de l'artère fémorale profonde dans le traitement de l'artérite femoro-poplitée et jambière. Chirurgie 97: 125–133

Hershey FB, Auer AI (1974) Extended surgical approach to the profunda femoris artery. Surg Gynecol Obstet 138: 88–90

Lawson DW, Gallico GG, Patton AS (1983) Limb salvage by extended profundaplasty of occluded deep femoral arteries. Am J Surg 145: 458–463

Leather RP, Shah DM, Karmody AM (1978) The use of extended profundaplasty in limb salvage. Am J Surg 136: 359–362

Leeds FH, Gilfillan RS (1961) Importance of profunda femoris artery in revascularization of ischemic limb. Arch Surg 82: 25–31

Martin P (1972) A reconsideration of arterial reconstruction below the inguinal ligament. J Cardiovasc Surg 13: 24–29

Martin P, Jamieson C (1974) The rationale for and measurement after profundaplasty. Surg Clin North Am 54: 95–109

Martin P, Renwick S, Stephenson C (1968) On the surgery of the profunda femoris artery. Br J Surg 55: 539–542

Martin P, Frawley JE, Barabas AP, Rosengarten DS (1972) On the surgery of atherosclerosis of the profunda femoris artery. Surgery 71: 182–189

Maurer PC, Lange J, Liepsch D (1979) Experimentelle Untersuchungen zur Stromungsdynamik im femoropoplitealen Bypass und in der A. profunda femoris (vor und nach Profundaplastik). In: Maurer PC, Fischer M, Scholz H (eds) Behandlungsgrundsatze der Chrirugie. Schattauer, Stuttgart, pp 367–377

Morris GC, Edwards WS, Cooley DA, Crawford ES, De Bakey ME (1961) Surgical importance of the profunda femoris artery. Analysis of 102 cases with combined aorto-iliac and femoro-popliteal occlusive disease treated by revascularization of deep femoral artery. Arch Surg 82: 32–37

Myhre HO (1977) The place of profundaplasty in surgical treatment of lower limb atherosclerosis. Acta Chir Scand 142: 105–108

Rollins DL, Towne JB, Bernhard VM, Baum PL (1985) Isolated profundaplasty for limb salvage. J Vasc Surg 2: 585–590

Schwilden E-D, van Dongen RJAM (1989) Surgery of the profunda femoris artery. In: Heberer G, van Dongen RJAM (eds) Vascular surgery. Springer, Berlin Heidelberg New York, pp 444–459

Strandness DE Jr (1970) Functional results after revascularization of the profunda femoris artery. Am J Surg 119: 240–245

Taylor LM, Baur GM, Eidemiller LR, Porter JM (1981) Extended profundaplasty. Indications and techniques with results of 46 procedures. Am J Surg 141: 539–542

Thompson BW, Read RC, Slayden JE, Boyd CM (1977) The role of primary and secondary profundaplasty in the treatment of vascular insufficiency. J Cardiovasc Surg 18: 55–62

Towne JB, Bernhard VM, Rollins DM, Baum PL (1981) Profundaplasty in perspective: limitations in the long-term management of limb ischemia. Surgery 90: 1037–46

Vaas F (1975) Some considerations concerning the deep femoral artery. Arch Chir Neerl 27: 25–34

van Dongen RJAM (1990) Profundaplastik – einst und jetzt. Angiol Arch 19: 88–92

van Dongen RJAM, Schwilden E-D (1974) Die Profundarevascularisation; alte und neue Methoden. Folia Angiol 22: 222–230

Waibel PP (1966) Autogenous reconstruction of the deep femoral artery. J Cardiovasc Surg 7: 179–181

Watelet J, Testart J, Teniere P, Chamoun S, Ducable G (1978) When can revascularization be limited to the profunda femoris alone? J Cardiovasc Surg 19: 345–354

10 Deep Femoral Artery Reconstruction

A.V. PERSSON and B. LANGE

The deep femoral artery (DFA) and superficial femoral artery (SFA) are the main outflow tracks used in reconstruction of the aortoiliac segment. The DFA can be used as an alternative source of inflow in arterial reconstruction in the lower limbs, particularly in reoperative procedures (Brewster et al. 1987; DePalma et al. 1980). Many patients who have ischemia that is severe enough to require bypass also have occlusion of the SFA. This occlusion usually begins at the adductor canal and may proceed up to the origin of the SFA. As a result, the SFA is the functional outflow even when the graft is attached to the common femoral artery (CFA). Therefore, the surgeon must visualize the orifice of the DFA at operation. When performing aortofemoral bypass for limb salvage, we often put a tongue of the distal aortofemoral bypass graft down onto the DFA. A DFA free of disease beyond the first centimeter will usually support an aortofemoral, axillary-to-femoral, or femoral-to-femoral graft even when the superficial femoral artery is entirely occluded. The distal end of the DFA has rich collaterals around the knee via the genicular arteries (see Fig. 6 in Chap. 1). In patients whose aortofemoral bypass has failed, the DFA is often the artery of choice to provide outflow. This chapter is limited to a discussion of reconstruction by grafting and endarterectomy of the DFA.

Limb Salvage

The goals of limb salvage are to eliminate rest pain, heal ischemic ulcers, and avoid major amputation or lower the amputation level. To achieve successful revascularization under these circumstances, flow to the groin must be adequate, i.e., the aortoiliac segment must be free of hemodynamically significant disease either naturally or by previously successful reconstruction. The primary method we use to determine how well the aortoiliac segment can support a graft is a noninvasive bidirectional continuous wave Doppler study to obtain a waveform of the CFA. Determining the status of the aortoiliac segment is important, because such a lesion is a common cause of failure of an otherwise perfect femoropopliteal artery bypass.

Direct revascularizazion with use of a distal bypass graft is the preferred treatment to attempt limb salvage in patients with multilevel infrainguinal disease. However, this technique may be impossible when it is associated with prohibitively high morbidity or mortality. Reconstruction of the DFA is a reasonable option under these circumstances. The most common situation in which this occurs is in patients with SFA occlusion accompanied by tight stenosis or occlusion of the DFA.

In the patient whose general medical condition or inadequate venous conduit precludes the performance of more distal reconstruction, the DFA may provide an adequate, although not perfect, outflow track. This can be accomplished by profundaplasty, distal endarterectomy, or bypass of the DFA beyond an occluded or significant stenosis. Control of rest pain, healing of ulcers, and avoidance of major amputation are possible when adequate collaterals exist around the knee (see Fig. 6 in Chap. 1). These may include either a patent popliteal artery (PA) with at least one open tibial vessel or extensive genicular arteries.

In most patients in whom the origin of the DFA is occluded, the proximal segment may not be usable, and dissection must proceed until a patent segment is found for the anastomosis. This dissection and anastomosis can almost always be carried out, except in the patient with advanced disease. The most common situation in which the proximal DFA is not usable but the distal vessel is adequate is in the patient who has had multiple procedures in the area.

The CFA and the proximal DFA are avoided completely, and the dissection is started more distally. The dissection must be carried out carefully because the branches are delicate and every one of them must be preserved. The branches are thin and act as the outflow track because the DFA is an end artery. The dissection can be carried down for 10–12 cm if necessary. Plastic vessel loops are used because they are gentler than metal clamps. The deep femoral vein is near the artery and often sends branches anteriorly and posteriorly. Thus, dissection is more difficult. When a previous dissection has been carried out, it is easy to enter fragile veins. When previous dissection has not been carried out, the vein can sometimes be used as a landmark to identify the artery. An intraoperative Doppler is useful in this regard because it is often easier to identify the vein than these low-velocity arteries. Several venous branches must often be sacrificed during the dissection to expose the artery sufficiently to create the anastomosis. Rarely can an end-to-end anastomosis be performed, because it is difficult to mobilize the artery in such a way as to construct the end-to-end anastomosis properly.

The length of the anastomosis is two to two and a half times the diameter of the DFA. This length usually provides a sufficient opening for adequate flow and a good angle between the graft and the DFA. The anastomosis is created using two sutures, starting one suture at each end of the arteriotomy. The position of the graft should be checked because it can become twisted whether the inflow is from the opposite femoral or the proximal iliac on the same side. Again, this is more of a problem in a repeat operation with much scarring than it is in a patient who is having the procedure performed for the first time.

Because many of the operations are repeat procedures, usually an artificial graft material, such as Dacron or polytetrafluoroethylene (PTFE) is chosen. Although we prefer Dacron, good results are possible with PTFE. How the graft is inserted rather than the graft material determines long-term patency. Results are usually good in patients who do not have diabetes because of the multiple geniculates and other collaterals that act as outflow. Patients who have diabetes usually have diseased geniculates, and such operations are associated with a low long-term patency rate, especially when the goal of the operation is to reperfuse the leg below the midcalf level. It is often more useful to provide increased flow to an above-the-knee or a below-the-knee amputation stump in patients who have diabetes than to save the limb.

In patients with nonreconstructable tibial or pedal disease associated with poor collaterals around the knee, the operative goals must be limited to lowering the amputation level, especially in older patients in whom the level of amputation is critically important in rehabilitation. Ambulation after digital, transmetatarsal, or below-the-knee amputation is better regardless of the age group. Above-the-knee amputation is associated with poor rehabilitation. A well-perfused DFA always ensures survival of an above-the-knee amputation stump. It will also, in most instances, provide enough flow for adequate healing of a below-the-knee amputation stump. Results after more distal amputation are less consistent, especially in patients with diabetes, who often have occlusive disease in the genicular arteries.

Inflow

The DFA can be used as an inflow vessel when outflow at the level of the knee or below is adequate to support a bypass graft. It is more common to select the DFA as the donor vessel at reoperation than it is to select it for the primary procedure. The CFA, if patent, may be a poor choice for anastomosis because of significant calcification, scarring, or groin infection. The DFA may also be chosen as the inflow vessel when a below-the-knee bypass is necessary, but adequate length of autologous vein is limited because of previous superficial phlebitis, previous revascularization, or coronary artery bypass.

Isolated Thigh Claudication

Buttock and thigh claudication are common in patients with atherosclerotic occlusive disease, particularly when the aortoiliac segment is involved. Buttock or thigh claudication without calf claudication is uncommon (Martin 1984). Buttock claudication is secondary to inadequate flow in the hypogastric arteries. Thigh claudication is caused by inadequate perfusion of the DFA. Occasionally, patients present with isolated thigh claudication. These patients usually have excellent inflow to the level of the CFA and a patent SFA with good blood flow below the knee. Such patients are symptomatic because the DFA is stenosed or occluded at its origin. This situation can occur in patients who have a functioning femoropopliteal artery bypass graft. In this instance, the pedal pulses will be palpable; however, thigh claudication will limit the patient's walking ability. This decreased perfusion of the DFA is caused by disease that was ignored at the time of the femoropopliteal bypass or has progressed since the time of operation.

In some cases, thigh claudication is due to disease isolated to the midportion of the DFA. This is not common, but is sometimes seen in patients who have had a successful popliteal bypass and a proximal profundaplasty.

Patients with neglected trauma to the DFA may present with similar symptoms. The trauma may have originated from a blunt object, a stab wound, or a low-velocity gun shot wound. In recent years, the most common cause is iatrogenic injuries associated with diagnostic and therapeutic procedures such as angiograms or balloon angioplasties of the coronary or distal leg vessels. These injuries are most commonly caused by procedures performed by cardiologists, because they use larger catheters for a prolonged period of time. Another source seen in inner city hospitals are patients who are intravenous (I.V.) drug addicts. These patients often use groin vessels as a site for injection of drugs. Such injections can cause injuries to any of the vessels in the groin including the DFA. These injuries are frequently associated with infection, which adds greatly to the challenge of the repair.

Reconstruction of stenosis of the mid-DFA is usually done by perfoming an endarterectomy and a patch angioplasty. Occasionally, the disease is so extensive that a bypass is necessary, but this is unusual. The patch can be vein or PTFE. If infection is present, one usually ligates the vessels if there is sufficient collateral. Once the infection has been resolved, a second operation is performed. This operation usually consists of a bypass to restore the arterial flow to the distal DFA. An endarterectomy cannot be performed under such conditions because of the intense scarring.

Pseudoaneurysms in the groin, secondary to arterial invasive procedures, are becoming more common. Although, occasionally, a patient will present with a gunshot or stab wound isolated to this area, the most common cause of trauma is iatrogenic (Rapoport et al. 1985). A busy cardiac service may perform one or two each month. They usually originate in the CFA and are controlled by using compression guided by the duplex Doppler scanning probe. This compression rarely works with pseudoaneurysms in the DFA. The DFA is deeper and below the fascia. This prevents adequate compression of the pseudoaneurysm, and in our experience these pseudoaneurysms must be closed by performing an open surgical procedure.

True Aneurysm

Of all of the abnormalities affecting the DFA, true aneurysm is probably the rarest, accounting for less than 0.5% of all peripheral arterial aneurysms (Flinn et al. 1982). Asymptomatic aneurysms are usually incidental findings noted during workup for other associated vascular problems and are particularly noticeable when the aneurysm is large and locally painful. It may be accompanied by a mass compressing an adjacent nerve or vein. Embolization or thrombosis with ischemia or rupture may occur, although the exact incidence of these complications is not known.

Management of DFA aneurysms consists of ligation or resection and reconstruction by grafting. Results of ligation have almost uniformly been poor, probably because these lesions occur in patients with significant arteriosclerotic vascular disease who are already at risk for ischemic complications. On the other hand, reconstruction by interposition or bypass grafts with autogenous vein or materials have been associated with favorable results in the few cases reported (Boren et al. 1980).

Preoperative Evaluation

Careful history taking and physical examination are of primary importance in the evaluation and treatment of patients with arterial disease. The severity of symptoms is often the determinant factor in assessing the need for aggressive therapy. Noninvasive arterial studies are performed next. Segmental pressure readings in conjunction with Doppler waveform analysis should be obtained routinely to determine the level and severity of disease. A systolic leg pressure that is 30% less than the systolic brachial pressure suggests the presence of stenosis or occlusion in the leg severe enough to force blood flow through an alternative higher-resistance system. The classic example of this situation is SFA occlusion in which the blood flow is diverted through the higher-resistance DFA system. If the ankle-to-brachial ratio and the waveform analysis suggest the presence of more than one lesion, the location of the additional disease must be determined. The source of the disease could be proximal (inflow), distal (outflow), or in the DFA. Normal results of waveform analysis in the CFA rule out proximal disease in the iliac artery. If waveforms in the popliteal and tibial vessels are abnormal but similar in severity, the secondary lesion is probably not in these vessels. In this situation, the presence of horizontal disease rather than vertical disease should be suspected, i.e., the secondary lesion may be in the origin of the DFA. Such disease can be documented with the use of the color Doppler scanner. In our experience, the DFA can be evaluated at its origin and distally for about 4–5 cm. The status of the DFA can also be documented at the time of angiography. Angiography is required in almost all patients undergoing arterial reconstruction of the lower limb. In patients with severe aortoiliac disease, the DFA may not be well delineated.

Patients with severe aortoiliac occlusive disease have such slow flow in the leg that standard arteriography does not adequately demonstrate the anatomy below the inguinal ligament. However,

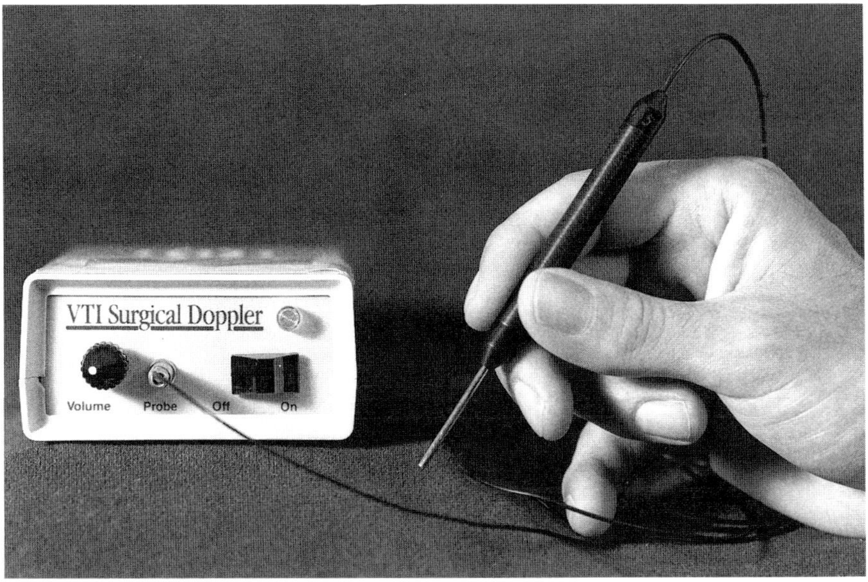

Fig. 1. Intraoperative Doppler Device with 30-MHz carrier frequency and a 2-mm Doppler crystal

we have been able to demonstrate patency of the DFA in these patients with the use of the color Doppler scanner. Determining the number of branch vessels present is useful when the DFA is dissected out to insert an aortofemoral graft or axillary bifemoral graft. In reoperative procedures, the groin is often extremely scarred, and knowledge of the expected anatomy of the patent vessels prevents unnecessary dissection. Interrogation with an intraoperative Doppler study is useful in localizing the patent artery at reoperation (Fig. 1).

Treatment

The two most common procedures performed on the DFA are bypass from the aorta and local angioplasty. Distal endarterectomy is occasionally indicated. Angioplasty is discussed in detail in Chap. 9.

Endarterectomy of the DFA distal to the orifice of occlusion is of value when no diffuse disease is present in the entire vessel (Nunez et al. 1988). Endarterectomy is also useful when the disease extends only for a few centimeters down the artery. Here, as

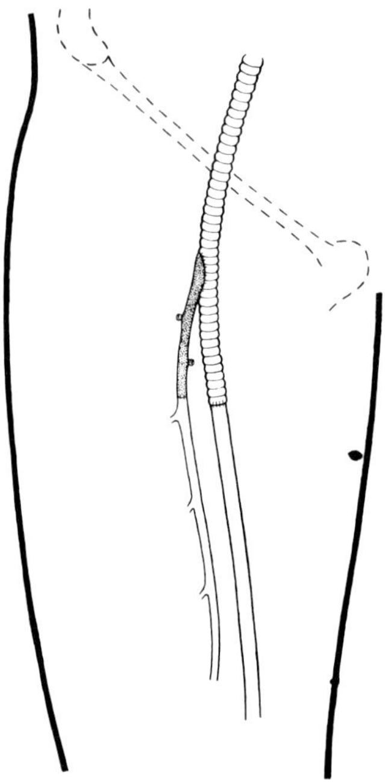

Fig. 2. Aortic-to-superficial femoral artery bypass graft. The proximal deep femoral artery (DFA) is replaced by an interposition vein graft. Printed by permission of the Lahey Clinic

elsewhere, the goal is to develop a plane in the outer media and remove all plaque until it feathers under direct vision. When the distal end of the plaque cannot be removed, it must be tacked down using 6–0 sutures. Tacking sutures are placed longitudinally, one through the endarterectomized segment and one through the plaque. To prevent the formation of a pleat, the sutures are placed in an interrupted fashion. A long tongue of the graft can be used to construct one wall of the endartectomized segment. When local endarterectomy of the distal vessel is being performed, the vessel will not close without the use of a patch. Although a PTFE graft can be used, the distal vessel is usually too small, and a segment of vein, preferably the distal saphenous vein at the medial malleolus, is used.

Reconstruction by interposition graft is appropriate when aneurysms in the CFA are resected and in the treatment of trauma (Sproul 1968). The most frequent indication for an interposition graft is in reoperative surgery when the CFA is the site of a previous arterial reconstructive procedure. In these patients, the proximal DFA is usually diseased just distal to the anastomosis. Segmental resection with interposition of autologous or synthetic graft material (Fig. 2) permits end-to-end anastomosis, which is hemodynamically better and seems to be associated with fewer problems related to intimal hyperplasia. Again, autologous vein is used because of the small diameter of these vessels.

Inflow Bypass Grafts

Use of the DFA as the outflow vessel in the management of patients with aortoiliac disease, regardless of the indication, is common. The inflow can be through the aorta (Brewster et al. 1987), contralateral CFA (Persson et al. 1980) (Fig. 3), axillary artery (Persson 1984) (Fig. 4), or iliac artery. These inflow sites lend themselves to primary reconstruction or reoperation. The distal DFA is particular useful when the groin is heavily scarred or is the site of previous infection (Fig. 5). In the patient who requires arterial reconstruction for limb salvage, thigh claudication, aneurysm, or trauma, bypass from the ipsilateral CFA may be the most efficacious therapy. A 6-mm or 8-mm Dacron graft is used in these patients. When only the DFA is available as a runoff vessel,

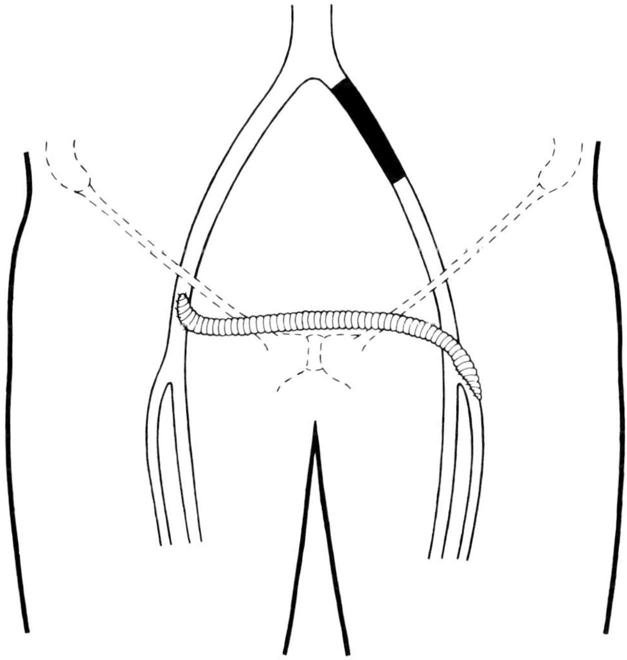

Fig. 3. Right to left femoral-to-femoral graft with distal end anastomosed to left deep femoral artery (DFA). Printed by permission of the Lahey Clinic

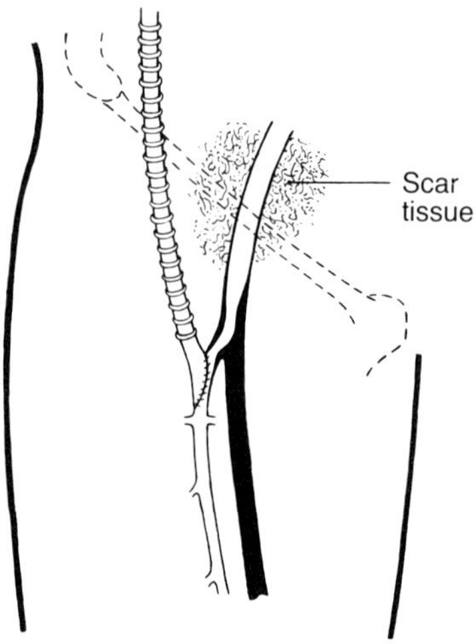

Fig. 4. Distal anastomosis in an axillary-to-deep femoral artery (DFA) bypass employing ringed polytetrafluoroethylene graft. Printed by permission of the Lahey Clinic

a 6-mm graft is used. Other surgeons prefer the use of PTFE or autologous vein (Rutherford and Bauer 1989).

Surgical Procedures

The standard approach to expose the DFA is an extension of the one used for the CFA. An S-shaped incision is made; the lateral aspect is just below the right iliac crest, and the medial aspect is over the saphenous vein (see Fig. 3 in Chap. 7). An incision that runs lateral to the artery so that the lymphatics can be rectracted medially causes less foot edema. The inguinal ligament is freed from the fascia, proving more exposure to the proximal CFA. After the CFA has been isolated, it can be followed distally to the origin of the SFA and the DFA. The DFA comes off in all directions: posterior, medial, and lateral to the SFA. It is exposed by proceeding anteriorly along the DFA. The vein passing over the anterior aspect of the DFA can be sacrificed. When further exposure is needed, the vessel is followed down into the thigh, with progressive retraction on the SFA and the transection of the overlying veins. Within the first 2–3 cm of its origin, usually one and commonly two major branches of the SFA are found. When the vessel is being used as an outflow tract, dissection beyond the first branch is rarely necessary (King et al. 1984). However, when it is being used as an inflow vessel, it usually must be dissected out for a distance of two or three branches.

Fig. 5. The deep femoral artery (DFA) is used as a source of inflow in a patient with an ischemic limb and scarred groin. Printed by permission of the Lahey Clinic

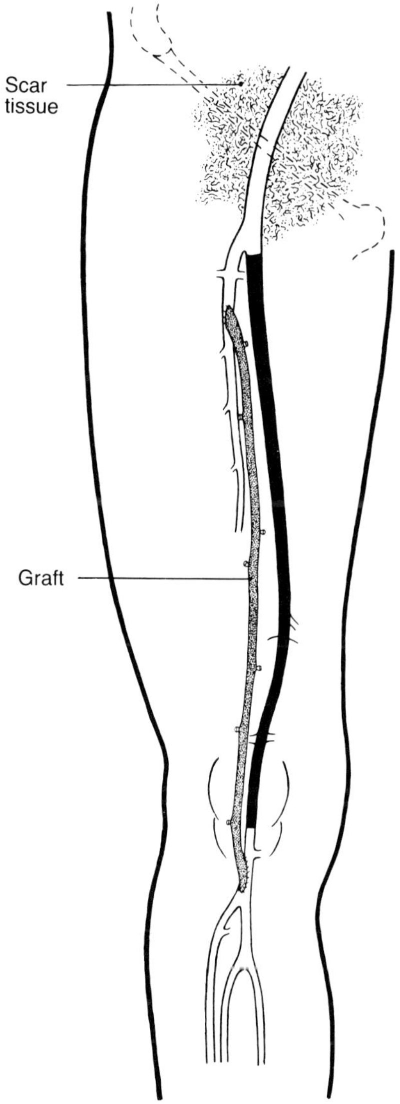

Graft Material

The choice of graft material conforms to the rules for others parts of the body. Vein or endarterectomized artery is the graft material of choice for using interposition or infrainguinal bypasses (Rollins et al. 1985a). A large-caliber PTFE or Dacron graft is appropriate for bypassing aortoiliac disease. A smaller-caliber synthetic vessel is an excellent choice for an interposition graft of short length. A synthetic graft that does not cross the knee joint is associated with a patency rate that approaches that for autologous material. Thus, such grafts are a reasonable choice, particularly in reoperative procedures. These grafts, like other grafts in the leg, will remain open if the blood flow velocity in the graft is high.

The proper choice of graft in the presence of infection is controversial. Unless it is impossible, autologous vein should be used. Some reports (Freischlag and Moore 1989) indicate that in the presence of infected pseudoaneurysms, a PTFE graft has worked satisfactorily as a patch. Autologous material is preferred when the graft is to be used as a conduit.

Exposed and infected graft material in the groin does not necessarily have to be removed. When this situation occurs, the infected native artery ruptures and not the graft itself. When the native artery is not exposed and weakened by infection, the wound may be allowed to heal by secondary intention, particularly when the patch only is involved. The anastomoses tend to be buried in the tissue and are not exposed to the surface. These patients should be observed carefully, usually in a hospital setting.

Type of Anastomosis

Intuitively, end-to-end anastomosis appears to be more consistent with laminar flow and less likely to develop turbulence and secondary disease. Evidence in support of this is seen daily in our laboratory where grafts are examined with a color Doppler scanner. Little or no turbulence is seen in an end-to-end anastomosis between the graft and the native artery of nearly equal size. Significant turbulence is seen when an end-to-side anastomosis is fashioned. As the angle becomes larger (approaches 90°), the turbulence increases. When an end-to-side anastomosis is constructed, placing the graft at an angle of approximately 30° to the native vessel provides the least turbulence (Fig. 6) and appears to be more important in an infrainguinal anastomosis than in an abdominal anastomosis. Studies (Brewster 1989) comparing end-to-side with end-to-end anastomosis in the proximal aorta have failed to reveal any difference in long-term patency. End-to-end anastomosis is performed when technically possible. When the proximal anastomosis is being created, flow cannot be sacrified in the vessel distal to the anastomosis, particularly when the DFA is used as the inflow vessel. Sacrificing flow into the thigh for the sake of a less turbulent anastomosis is inappropriate.

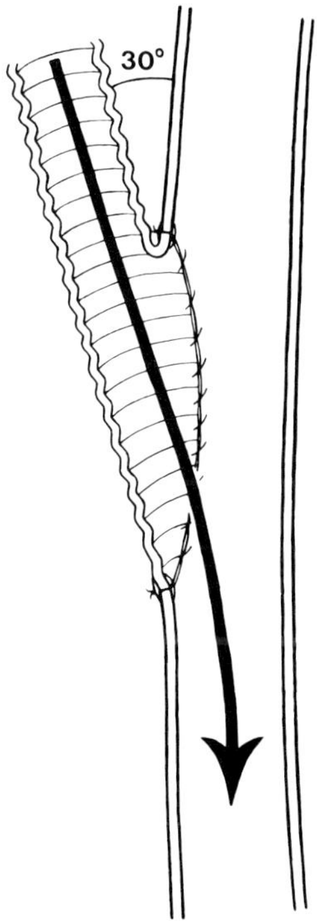

Fig. 6. End-to-side anastomosis is placed at an angle not greater than 30° to the recipient vessel. Printed by permission of the Lahey Clinic

Suture Material

In the past, vascular anastomoses were created using interrupted silk sutures. However, deterioration of the silk over time and subsequent pseudoaneurysm formation stimulated a search for a new suture material that could last indefinitely. Monofilament polypropylene sutures and braided Ti-Cron sutures have met these needs. The decision to use one material or the other is dependent on the personal preference of the surgeon. No good evidence is available to prove that one type is superior to the other. A running suture is more commonly used than multiple interrupted sutures. When a continuous suture is being placed, use of monofilament material has the theoretical advantage of tending to be more slippery. Also, the surgeon can adjust the tension uniformly during suturing. However, when the suture is pulled too tightly, the caliber of the anastomosis can be reduced by the "purse string" effect.

A multifilament PTFE suture has recently been introduced, but we have had no personal experience with this material. It is too early to comment on or to predict whether its long-term durability is comparable to that obtained with the suture material we have been using with success for the last decade. It is possible that this suture material will hold up as well, as grafts made of the same material have stood the test of time.

Use of Anticoagulants

Except in the case of specifically identified hypercoagulable states, antiplatelet agents and anticoagulants are usually not of short-term or long-term benefit. The one possible exception is in a graft presenting a low flow rate (Bandyk 1990), particularly an infrainguinal graft that crosses the knee. Our experience echoes that reported in the literature.

We give 5000 U heparin intravenously before cross-clamping and supplement the dose with 2000 U every hour. In obese patients or in patients in whom a clot is developing in the wound, the dose in supplemented further. If low velocity is noted in the graft after operation and no correctable lesion is evident on postoperative angiography, the patient is deep in a heparinized state postoperatively. The medication is changed to crystalline sodium warfarin (Coumadin), maintaining a low dose. In the postoperative period, the peak systolic velocity is measured at the midgraft level using the new color Doppler scanner. If the peak velocity is less than 40 cm/s, the graft is classified as threatened. Grafts with a velocity greater than 60 cm/s usually remain patent. We have adopted the policy described by Bandyk (1990): a therapeutic regimen of low-dose Coumadin is begun in any patient with a graft peak velocity of less than 60 cm/s at the midgraft level unless a definite contraindication to Coumadin exists.

Intraoperative Assessment

Palpation is useful method for predicting the success of a graft. When the upstroke of the pulse is equal to the downstroke, the inflow is presumably equal to the outflow. However, when the upstroke is longer, an inflow problem should be suspected. In the case of a longer downstroke, the outflow should be assessed. This can be performed either with the examiner's finger or, more precisely, with an intraoperative Doppler study and printout. Another advantage of an intraoperative Doppler study is that if it is performed approximately 60° to the flow in the graft, a reproducible velocity can be obtained. Although this is subjective, the examiner can soon begin to recognize, either audibly or visually, a "good" velocity from a "bad" velocity. If reverse flow is demonstrated during diastole, an excellent flow and a good prognosis are ensured. Reverse flow in diastole occurs only when laminar flow is present. The presence of turbulence prevents the occurrence of reverse flow. Therefore, Doppler sampling should be obtained at the midgraft level and not near the anastomoses.

Intraoperative angiography is performed on all patients with infrainguinal arterial bypass grafts. Two views are obtained: one with the proximal artery clamped and one with the vessel wide open. Intraoperative performance of arteriography has several advantages. It permits the identification of a technical error that can be corrected at operation. The runoff can be assessed more accurately and the long-term success predicted. The onset of postoperative failure may only by prevented by devising a better means for runoff. In many instances, this will prevent unnecessary reexploration and futile attempts at salvage.

A standard marker is placed beside the graft to help determine the size of the vessels intraoperatively, to delineate the anatomy, and to aid in planning subsequent surgical treatment. It also provides a standard for comparison with the color ultrasonic images.

Results

The success of the treatment of arterial vascular disease is measured by the functional capacity of the patient and patency of the arterial reconstruction. When the DFA is used as the only outflow vessel in the treatment of patients with aortoiliac disease, the 5-year patency rate is excellent (Simma et al. 1986). In many series (Towne et al. 1981; Rollins et al. 1985b; Miksic and Novak 1986), when the DFA is used alone, results are comparable to those when the DFA and the SFA are both used. The patency rate at 5 years is 90% for aortobifemoral artery grafts and 80% for unilateral aortoiliac or femoral-to-femoral grafts (Welsh and Repetto 1975). The rate of limb loss in patients who present with claudication is less than 5% at 5 years. The functional result is better than the primary patency rate.

The success rate is more difficult to determine when the DFA is used as an outflow vessel or as an inflow vessel in patients with limb salvage (Rollins et al. 1985b; Ouriel et al. 1987). These cases are reported in different ways. Preoperative patient selection affects the outcome greatly. Results of revascularization in patients with limb salvage are similar regardless of whether it is the first or second procedure. In one study (Brief et al. 1975), the overall 5-year patency rate was 76% for femoral-to-femoral bypass and was 96% for aortofemoral bypass grafts. Their rate in axillary-to-DFA grafts was only 26% at 5 years. The overall amputation rate was 20%; 82% of the patients had relief of rest pain, and 71% had complete resolution of claudication. A decrease in the amputation rate is often difficult to assess. Most reports (Rollins et al. 1985b) suggest that the amputation rate is lowered when a graft to the DFA is successful. However, no good randomized study has been performed. Studies to date are a comparison of what the surgeon predicted would happen with what in fact did happen after the operation. Healing of ischemic ulcers and relief of rest pain are similarly difficult to assess, although indications of improvement are much more objective because rest pain rarely resolves spontaneously.

In all of these patients, the status of the distal vascular bed is the most important prognostic factor. In one study (Ouriel et al. 1987), when the popliteal segment was open, 90% of patients had symptomatic improvement. When it was occluded, only 30% of patients had improvement. Similarly, when the profundapopliteal collateral index was less than 0.25, 85% of patients had improvement, but when it was greater than 0.25, only 20% of patients had improvement (Ouriel et al. 1987).

In patients with isolated thigh claudication, symptom resolution and patency rates appear to be high; however, only small series and case reports are reported in the literature (Towne et al. 1981). In patients with previously distal bypass and few knee collaterals, outcome is reported in relationship to limb salvage rather than resolution of symptoms. The true success rate is difficult to document in the literature.

Reports of the results of DFA reconstruction for atherosclerotic aneurysm are similarly sparse, but the results appear to parallel those of repair of the same condition in the PA. Of course, resolution of symptoms related to local compression of veins and nerves accompanies repair. However, results after the development of emboli from the aneurysm or thrombosis or rupture are less satisfying. Distal emboli may result in subclinical loss of distal DFA branches, which, after thrombosis, can progress to significant thigh muscle necrosis. This is especially true in patients with preexisting SFA occlusion. Distal emboli can also produce limb-threatening distal ischemia analogous to that seen in graft thrombosis caused by a DFA stricture. Repair in these settings is still associated with a 20% amputation rate.

For the same reasons, a ruptured aneurysm is associated with a similar prognosis. Ligation is only an option when the SFA is open and results are good. However, when the DFA is the only outflow vessel from the groin, reconstruction is mandatory but still results in a significant amputation rate, chiefly because of the profound ischemia at presentation.

Success in the treatment of traumatic lesions of the DFA would seem to be a function of preexisting arteriosclerotic vascular disease. During World War II, the Korean War, and the Vietnam War, simple ligation in the few reported cases of DFA trauma occurring in otherwise healthy young men was not associated with any amputations. Different results would have been expected if these patients had had a significant preexisting vascular disease, specifically SFA occlusion, but no evidence of this can be found in the literature.

Results of repair of the complications of trauma, including pseudoaneurysm in the DFA, would be expected to parallel the initial treatment of hemorrhage or expanding hematoma. An exception to this may occur in large DFA with significant associated proximal arterial aneurysmal change and venous dilation, but, again, no series has reported specifically on this problem.

Conclusions

Use of the DFA as an outflow vessel in procedures for aortoiliac disease or as an inflow vessel in infrainguinal bypass for limb salvage is clearly as good as use of either CFA or SFA. The same cannot be said for the use of DFA instead of a femoropopliteal bypass. In this setting, which is usually desperate because of the lack of adequate distal vasculature, the presence of infection, or general debility of the patient, use of the DFA is a reasonable choicc and offers significant improvement in limb salvage. The outcome of repair of atherosclerotic aneurysm in the DFA, especially when associated with other significant atherosclerosis, specifically SFA occlusion, is somewhere in between. In the treatment of trauma to the DFA and its complications, the results are good without preexisting atherosclerosis.

Good patient selection using noninvasive and arteriographic criteria, meticulous intraoperative technique, and close postoperative follow-up procedures result in the highest patency and limb salvage rates.

References

Bandyk DF (1990) Postoperative surveillance of infrainguinal bypass. Surg Clin North Am 70: 71–85

Boren CH, Towne JB, Bernhard VM, Salles-Cunha S (1980) Profundapopliteal collateral index: a guide to successful profundaplasty. Arch Surg 115: 1366–1372

Brewster DC (1989) Direct reconstruction for aortoiliac occlusive disease. In: Rutherford RB (ed) Vascular surgery, 3rd edn. Saunders, Philadelphia, pp 667–691

Brewster DC, Meier GH III, Darling RC, Moncure AC, LaMuraglia GM, Abbott WM (1987) Reoperation for aortofemoral graft limb occlusion: optimal methods and long term results. J Vasc Surg 5: 363–374

Brief DK, Brener BJ, Alpert J, Parsonnet V (1975) Crossover femorofemoral grafts followed up five years or more: an analysis. Arch Surg 110: 1294–1299

DePalma RG, Malgieri JJ, Rhodes RS, Clowes AW (1980) Profunda femoris bypass for secondary revascularization. Surg Gynecol Obstet 151: 387–390

Flinn WR, Yao JST, Bergan JJ (1982) Aneurysms of secondary and tertiary branches of major arteries. In: Began JJ, Yao JST (eds) Aneurysms: diagnosis and treatment. Grune and Stratton, New York, pp 449–467

Freischlag JA, Moore WS (1989) Infection in prosthetic grafts. In: Rutherford RB (ed) Vascular surgery, 3rd edn. Saunders, Philadelphia, pp 510–521

King TA, DePalma RG, Rhodes RS (1984) Diabetes mellitus and atherosclerotic involvement of the profunda femoris artery. Surg Gynecol Obstet 159: 553–556

Martin RS III (1984) Thigh claudication due to profunda femoris artery occlusion. J Vasc Surg 1: 692–694

Miksic K, Novak B (1986) Profunda femoris revascularization in limb salvage. J Cardiovasc Surg 27: 544–552

Nunez AA, Veith FJ, Collier P, Ascer A, White Flores S, Gupta SK (1988) Direct approaches to the distal portions of the deep femoral artery for limb salvage bypasses. J Vasc Surg 8: 576–581

Ouriel K, DeWeese JA, Ricotta JJ, Green RM (1987) Revascularization of the distal profunda femoris artery in the reconstructive treatment of aortoiliac occlusive disease. J Vasc Surg 6: 217–220

Persson AV (1984) Extra-anatomic bypass for lower extremity revascularization. In: Rutherford RB (ed) Vascular surgery, 2nd edn. Saunders, Philadelphia, pp 523–526

Persson AV, Dyer VE, West LS (1980) Femoral-to-femoral bypass graft. Surg Clin North Am 60: 537–544

Rapoport S, Sniderman KW, Morse SS, Proto MH, Ross GR (1985) Pseudoaneurysm: a complication of faulty technique in femoral arterial puncture. Radiology 154: 529–530

Rollins DL, Towne JB, Bernhard VM, Baum PL (1985a) Endarterectomized superficial femoral artery as an arterial patch. Arch Surg 120: 367–369

Rollins DL, Towne JB, Bernhard VM, Baum PL (1985b) Isolated profundaplasty for limb salvage. J Vasc Surg 2: 585–590

Rutherford RB, Bauer AE (1989) Extra-anatomic bypass. In Rutherford RB (ed) Vascular surgery, 3rd edn. Saunders, Philadelphia, pp 705–716

Simma W, Bassiouny H, Hartl P, Brcke P (1986) Evaluation of profundoplasty in reconstructions of combined aorto-iliac and femoro-popliteal occlusive disease. J Cardiovasc Surg 27: 141–145

Sproul G (1968) Reconstruction of the profunda femoris artery. Surgery 63: 871–874

Towne JB, Bernhard VM, Rollins DL, Baum PL (1981) Profundaplasty in perspective: limitations in the long-term management of limb ischemia. Surgery 90: 1037–1046

Welsh P, Repetto R (1975) Revascularization of the profunda femoris artery in aortoiliac occlusive disease. Surgery 78: 389–393

11 Follow-Up Studies and Conclusions

M. DUSMET

Most procedures for lower-limb ischemia involve the iliosuperficial femoral axis. However, in a small but significant number of patients who have often undergone one or more reconstructive procedures, an alternative approach is required. The deep femoral artery (DFA) can be an ideal relatively disease-free site for anastomosis in the management of these difficult patients. In proximal procedures the DFA can provide sufficient runoff to maintain patency providing it has a well-developed collateral network and a patent popliteal artery (PA) with at least one good crural artery. Under these conditions ischemic lesions will heal and claudication can be completely relieved. In distal bypasses a healthy DFA can offer an alternative source of inflow. This is particularly useful in two circumstances: when the groin is heavily scarred by previous operations or is infected, and when a more distal site is required for a venous femorodistal bypass and only a short amount of vein is available. Finally, as described in detail by van Dongen (Chap. 9), profundaplasty can be a precious limb-saving operation in carefully selected patients.

In this chapter, I will not try to summarize the indications and results of all the procedures involving the DFA. This has been done throughout the book. As in all fields of surgery, if the indications and above all the contraindications are respected, the results are quite good. Use of the DFA can provide limb salvage and relief of symptoms in a large majority of patients where indicated, even if these techniques apply only to a minority. In La Chaux-de-Fonds (Switzerland; head surgeon, Dr. M. Merlini) we have used these techniques in exactly 10% of procedures for lower-limb ischemia with excellent results. It is impossible to say how many limbs were salvaged, but we were impressed by the number of completely asymptomatic patients (seven out of 14, i.e., 50%) with a mean follow-up of 21 months (13 out of 19 patients presented with critical limb ischemia).

Follow-Up Studies

There is little or no literature on the follow-up of procedures using the DFA, but it seems logical to apply what is known about standard procedures for lower-limb ischemia. It is said that obstructions due to technical faults, infection, and hypercoagulability occur during the first 30 days and that thereafter occlusions are due to disease progression in the native artery above or below the graft or to graft stenosis (Bandyk 1990). Approximately 20%–30% of femorodistal procedures will occlude during the first postoperative year or two (Berkowitz et al. 1992; Brennan et al. 1991). Furthermore, roughly 60%–70% of all graft occlusions occur during the first 12–18 months and only around 20% after the first 2–3 years (Mills et al. 1993; Grigg et al. 1988; Sanchez et al. 1991).

Finally, most authors agree that revision of a failing graft gives better results than intervention on a failed graft, improving patency rates by as much as 20%–50% (Bandyk et al. 1991; Mattos et al. 1993; Killewich et al. 1990; Mills et al. 1990). This is the rationale for most graft surveillance programs. The most common sequence is a first visit at 4–6 weeks postoperatively, then at 3, 6, 9, and 12 months. If at that point nothing alarming has been seen, patients should be followed every 3–6 months for the second year, and it is probably useful to see patients every 6 months beyond the 2-year mark for those 20% still at risk (Bandyk 1990; Berkowitz et al. 1992; Mills et al. 1993; Idu et al. 1993; Green et al. 1990).

The first follow-up examination is the on-table completion angiogram as well as on-table hemodynamic assessment (Bandyk et al. 1991; Bandyk et al. 1989). This will allow technical faults to be seen and corrected at once and as well as a precise determination of the number and patency of outflow vessels. In distal bypasses the number of patent pedal arches (anterior and/or posterior) can be a good determinant of prognosis: when one is intact in high procedures or both in low ones, the patency rate was 81% at 6 months, but when this was not the case all grafts occluded (Karacagil et al. 1990). For above-the-knee procedures the number and quality of the crural arteries is determinant.

Some authors prefer to perform completion angioscopy. This technique is probably advantageous for optimal preparation of the in situ venous graft and as good as angiography for the detection of technical faults needing immediate correction, but it cannot evaluate the runoff (Miller et al. 1993; Baxter et al. 1990). On balance, angioscopy is probably as good or better for in situ venous grafting, but angiography is preferable for all other techniques. Doing both is too cumbersome, time-consuming, and expensive to propose outside the setting of a prospective study comparing both methods.

Perioperative graft flow velocity (GFV) measurements can also be useful. A flow of less than 40 cm/s indicates a high risk of occlusion, whereas a GFV of over 60 cm/s presents a very low risk. When the on-table peak systolic flow velocity is lower than 40 cm/s in the smallest segment of the graft, especially if there is no forward diastolic flow, then a thorough search for a technical error is mandatory (Bandyk et al. 1989).

As alluded to throughout the book, a certain number of DFA procedures, especially profundaplasties, are done as "last ditch" attempts at limb salvage in frail patients. In certain cases the only objective is to lower the amputation level from above to below the knee. When all the pre- and perioperative data indicate that no further vascular procedures (including lumbar sympathectomy) can reasonably be proposed, then I do not think that it is sensible or useful to ask these patients to come back for scheduled follow-up unless they are part of a prospective study. It can be expensive and difficult for these patients to come, they cause extra demands on the vascular laboratory staff, and the patients will derive no benefit from the follow-up. On the other hand, all other patients should be aggressively assessed on a regular basis. Most of these patients have already undergone previous procedures, and sometimes salvaging a failing graft will make all the difference between continuing relief of symptoms and amputation.

What Should Be Done at Each Follow-Up Visit?

The ideal follow-up visit would be cost effective and noninvasive, would detect all failing grafts, and would be short and simple to perform. Unfortunately, these goals are to a certain extent mutually exclusive. The undisputable gold standard of graft permeability and stenosis (which can also occur in the native inflow and outflow vessels) is angiography. This is too invasive and too expensive to perform on a routine basis at each visit (Mills et al. 1993; Idu et al. 1992). All other techniques have basically been developed to triage patients for angiography, although some surgeons operate on the basis of the duplex examination alone (Bandyk et al. 1991).

Each patient should undergo clinical assessment (severity of symptoms, rest pain, ischemic lesions, presence or absence of palpable pulses and/or bruits). This clinical evaluation has a very low sensitivity for detecting failing grafts (Bandyk 1990; Bandyk et al. 1991). However, Sanchez et al. (1991) detected 150 failing grafts (2187 procedures; 7%) on clinical examination alone.

Ankle–Brachial Indexes

Just about everything has been written about the sensitivity of the ankle–brachial index (ABI) for detecting failing grafts. While it is undoubtedly true that the ABI is not the "gold standard" for the diagnosis of a failing vein graft, the technique can give very good results if carefully applied. Furthermore, not all vascular surgeons have a well-staffed vascular laboratory at their disposal that can perform duplex scans on all their patients at each follow-up visit. The ABI cannot be used in approximately 15%–20% of patients (who are often diabetic), because they have incompressible crural arteries (Idu et al. 1991). Thus when these patients ("best" ABI >1.3) are excluded, most, if not all, failing grafts can be detected by a drop in the resting ABI of >0.1 (Brennan et al. 1991; Green et al. 1990; Stierli et al. 1992). In fact, in one study (Stierli et al. 1992) two grafts at risk were detected by a fall in ABI of >0.1, whereas duplex examination was negative. Results are better if a stress test is added – ideally walking on a treadmill (10% slope at 4 km/h; Brennan et al. 1991; Wyatt et al. 1990). Again, a fall in the ABI of 0.1 can indicate a failing graft. However, only 50% of these frail patients, who often have healing lesions, serious disease of the other limb, or other limiting factors, can perform this test. An occlusive cuff inflated to 50 mmHg above systolic pressure produces the same fall in pressure, but can be performed in around 85% of patients (Wyatt et al. 1990). If the peak systolic flow velocity (PSFV) is measured by duplex scanning (PSFV <40 cm/s or >120 cm/s), this adds a prognostic indicator: when there is a fall in ABI without a PSFV of either less than 40 cm/s or more than 120 cm/s, then the incidence of sudden graft occlusion in the next 3 months is negligible. However, when both the ABI falls and the PSFV is outside these values, 66% of grafts occluded in the next 3 months (Green et al. 1990), although this was not verified by Mattos et al. (1993).

A fall of the ABI of only 0.10 will yield a substantial number of false-positive results, but requiring a fall of 0.15–0.20 is too insensitive (too many failed grafts). In one study where 15 out of 18 failing grafts had a fall of the ABI of >0.1, only 40% would have been detected if a fall of 0.2 had been required (Brennan et al. 1991). Similarly (Bandyk et al. 1989), in another study all 56 patients with failing grafts had a fall in ABI of >0.1 (mean, 0.24; range, 0.1–0.55), but only 38% showed a fall of >0.2.

Duplex Scanning

Duplex scanning is undoubtedly a very good method of graft surveillance. It can detect as many as 90%–100% of failing grafts, can reliably assess the degree of stenosis, and can measure flow rates. Entire grafts can usually be completely scanned, especially the subcutaneous in situ ones. Screening can be reliably done by measuring PSFV at set points of the graft and at the anastomotic areas (Mills et al. 1990, 1993) or by scanning the whole graft. Conventional and color scans give comparable results (Killewich et al. 1990), but the color scans can be simpler and shorter to perform; however, the equipment is more expensive (Idu et al. 1992; Stierli et al. 1992). A PSFV of <40–45 cm/s or >110–140 cm/s is highly indicative of stenosis or impending failure due to disease progression in the native arteries (Bandyk 1990; Mills et al. 1990, 1993; Idu et al. 1992; Buth et al. 1991). However, both Mattos et al. (1993) and Chang et al. (1990) did not find a PSFV <45 cm/s to be a reliable indicator of stenosis. A ratio of the maximal PSFV to that of an adjacent segment indicates a moderate stenosis when greater than 1.5. Some authors reverse this ratio (Grigg et al. 1988; Idu et al. 1993; Idu et al. 1992; Buth et al. 1991). A velocity ratio of >2 indicates a stenosis of more than 50% (Buth et al. 1991). Comparison of the PSFV to the previously recorded value is also very useful: when the PSFV falls by more than 30 cm/s between two follow-up visits, this indicates the presence of a hemodynamically significant stenosis (Bandyk et al. 1989, 1991). An increase in end-diastolic velocity (>20 cm/s) is indicative of more severe stenosis (>70%; Buth et al. 1991).

According to Bandyk et al. (1990), systolic spectral broadening with no increase in PSFV indicates a stenosis of >20%. When the stenosis is 20%–49%, the PSFV increases by 30% relative to a more proximal site and there is spectral broadening throughout the cycle, but the PSFV is <125 cm/s. When the stenosis is 50%–75%, the PSFV ratio rises to 2 (relative to a proximal segment) and the

PSFV is >125 cm/s. When the stenosis is greater than 75% there is, in addition, an end-diastolic velocity of >100 cm/s.

These examinations can be very time-consuming, can be operator dependent, and can fail to detect some stenosis, especially around the distal PA and the peroneal vessels (Bandyk 1990; Mills et al. 1993; Stierli et al. 1992; Wyatt et al. 1991).

Finally, waveform analysis can be useful: transformation of a triphasic to a monophasic or biphasic configuration in association with a decreased PSFV reliably predicted remote lesions in one author's experience (Bandyk 1990; Bandyk et al. 1989).

Impedance Analysis

Wyatt et al. (1991) described a computer-assisted analysis of Doppler waveforms and pulse volume recordings. Whether this is truly a measurement of impedance is a moot point (Wyatt et al. 1991). What is interesting is that the method was able to detect 20 out of 22 stenoses in the validation study and 33 out of 34 in the graft surveillance program when the impedance score was >0.45. All patients in the validation study underwent biplanar intra-arterial digital substraction angiography, whereas all patients in the surveillance program also had ABI measured and duplex scans. The method is simple and straightforward, noninvasive, and repeatable. If further studies from other centers can confirm these promising results, this could conceivably become the future gold standard of graft surveillance.

Recommendations

In light of all the above it seems that a reasonable option for graft surveillance would be a follow-up visit at 6 weeks and 3, 6, 9, 12, 15, 18, and 24 months after the operation and then every 6 months. At each visit, recurrent symptoms must be sought and a careful clinical examination performed. Any clinical deterioration in itself warrants aggressive examination of the graft, at least by complete duplex scanning and often by angiography. Unfortunately, clinical deterioration often heralds graft failure rather than a failing graft (Mills et al. 1990, 1993). If the clinical examination is unchanged and if the crural arteries are compressible, then the ABI should be measured at rest and after some form of stress testing (a 2-min walk on a treadmill or cuff occlusion). If in either circumstance the ABI falls more than 0.1, then duplex scanning is warranted, or at the very least the PSFV should be measured. If this is below 45 cm/s or greater than 110 cm/s, angiography should be performed.

Bandyk's criteria for graft revision (Bandyk et al. 1991) are pretty much endorsed by most authors. They include: (a) symptomatic limb ischemia, (b) hemodynamic deterioration in graft blood flow (a decrease in PSFV of more than 30 cm/s since the last visit or a fall in the ABI of >0.15), (c) low flow in the distal segment (PSFV <45 cm/s), and (d) a correctable occlusive lesion detected by duplex scanning or angiography (stenosis >75%). When "less" than this is found, close follow-up is warranted and when one of the above criteria is ultimately met then revision is recommended. Mattos et al. (1993) also found that stenoses of less than 50% tend to have a relatively benign outcome, as did Idu et al. (1992).

This proposal will obviously have to be adapted to each center's resources and capabilities. Many authors feel that duplex scanning is the best screening method, but the equipment is expensive and the examination can be time-consuming. Therefore, this is not a viable option in many centers for budgetary reasons. Careful monitoring by clinical examination and ABI measurement could be used to screen patients for duplex scanning. Patients with a stenosis of more than 50% as determined by duplex scanning could then undergo angiography and, if possible, the lesions could be treated by percutaneous transluminal angioplasty (Berkowitz et al. 1992; Sanchez et al. 1991) or any of a variety of procedures (excision/suture of a stenosis, vein patch angioplasty, short interposition vein graft, jump graft to a more distal patent artery etc.). If at this point it is determined that nothing more can be done, it might seem reasonable to stop following the patient on a regular basis (unless part of a research protocol). This often occurs because of distal disease progession. When the PSFV is less than 45 cm/s and no correctable lesions are identifiable, most grafts will occlude during the following 3–9 months (Bandyk et al. 1989). It is possible that long-term oral anticoagulation could improve this dismal outcome (Bandyk 1990; Kretschmer et al. 1992). If, however, some sort of procedure is performed, the patient starts the surveillance program with visits at 6 weeks and 3, 6, 9, 12, 15, and 18 months and then every 6 months.

When graft thrombosis occurs between follow-up visits, several authors recommend thrombolysis, then duplex scanning or angiography to try to detect a correctable lesion (Mills et al. 1993).

This proposal for graft surveillance is an empirical effort to provide cost- and resource-effective graft surveillance on the basis of the available data. Its value needs to be proven by a randomized prospective study.

Conclusions

The DFA is often used to provide outflow for proximal reconstructions when the superficial femoral artery (SFA) is occluded. It can also offer a precious alternative as a source of inflow for distal bypasses, especially in patients who have already undergone previous procedures that have failed. These procedures can avoid amputation for many patients, often with relief of symptoms of limb ischemia. In some patients, however, all that can be achieved is lowering the level of amputation from above to below the knee. However, even this is a worthwhile goal. Choosing the optimal level of amputation can be aided by measurement of the transcutaneous oxygen pressure (Bacharach et al. 1992).

As in all vascular procedures, postoperative surveillance is "all part of the service" (Harris 1992). Early recognition of failing grafts and aggressive intervention can improve patency rates by as much as 50%, and this is particularly important in these high-risk patients who have often had more or less all their veins used and for whom graft thrombosis can be particularly ominous.

References

Bacharach JM, Rooke TW, Osmundson PJ, Gloviczki P (1992) Predictive value of transcutaneous oxygen pressure and amputation success by use of supine and elevation measurements. J Vasc Surg 15: 558–563

Bandyk DF (1990) Postoperative surveillance of infrainguinal bypass. Surg Clin North Am 70: 71–85

Bandyk DF, Schmitt DD, Seabrook GR, Adams MB, Towne JB (1989) Monitoring functional patency of in situ saphenous vein bypasses: the impact of a surveillance protocol and elective revision. J Vasc Surg 9: 286–296

Bandyk DF, Bergamini TM, Towne JB, Schmitt DD, Seabrook GR (1991) Durability of vein graft revision: the outcome of secondary procedures. J Vasc Surg 13: 200–210

Baxter BT, Rizzo RJ, Flinn WR, Almgren CN, McCarthy WJ, Pearce WH, Yao JST (1990) A comparative study of intra-operative angioscopy and completion arteriography following femorodistal bypass. Arch Surg 125: 997–1002

Berkowitz HD, Fox AD, Deaton DH (1992) Reversed vein graft stenosis: early diagnosis and management. J Vasc Surg 15: 130–142

Brennan JA, Walsh AKM, Beard JD, Bolia AA, Bell PRF (1991) The role of simple non-invasive testing in infra-inguinal vein graft surveillance. Eur J Vasc Surg 5: 13–17

Buth J, Disselhoff B, Sommeling C, Stam L (1991) Color-flow duplex criteria for grading stenosis in infrainguinal vein grafts. J Vasc Surg 14: 716–728

Chang BB, Leather RP, Kaufman JL, Kupinski AM, Leopold PW, Shah DM (1990) Hemodynamic characteristics of failing infrainguinal in situ vein bypass. J Vasc Surg 12: 596–600

Green RM, McNamara J, Ouriel K, DeWeese JA (1990) Comparison of infrainguinal graft surveillance techniques. J Vasc Surg 11: 207–215

Grigg MJ, Nicolaides AN, Wolfe JHN (1988) Femorodistal vein bypass graft stenosis. Br J Surg 75: 737–740

Harris PL (1992) Vein graft surveillance – all part of the service. Br J Surg 79: 97–98

Idu MM, Truyen E, Buth J (1992) Surveillance of lower extremity vein grafts. Eur J Vasc Surg 6: 456–462

Idu MM, Blankenstein JD, de Gier P, Truyen E, Buth J (1993) Impact of a color-flow duplex surveillance program on infrainguinal vein graft patency: a five-year experience. J Vasc Surg 17: 42–53

Karacagil S, Almgren B, Bowald S, Eriksson I (1990) A new method of angiographic runoff evaluation in femorodistal reconstructions. Significant correlation with early graft patency. Arch Surg 125: 1055–1058

Killewich LA, Fischer C, Bartlett ST (1990) Surveillance of in situ infrainguinal bypass grafts: conventional vs. color flow duplex ultrasonography. J Cardiovasc Surg 31: 662–667

Kretschmer G, Herbst F, Prager M, Sautner T, Wenzl E, Berlakovich GA, Zekert F, Marosi L, Schemper M (1992) A decade of oral anticoagulant treatment to maintain antologous vein grafts for femoropopliteal atherosclerosis. Arch Surg 127: 1112–1115

Mattos MA, van Bemmelen PS, Hodgson KJ, Ramsey DE, Barkmeier LD, Sumner DS (1993) Does correction of stenoses identified with color duplex scanning improve infrainguinal graft patency? J Vasc Surg 17: 54–66

Miller A, Marcaccio EJ, Tannenbaum GA, Kwolek CJ, Stonebridge PA, Lavin PT, Gibbons GW, Pomposelli FB, Freeman DV, Campbell DR, LoGerfo FW (1993) Comparison of angioscopy and angiography for monitoring infrainguinal bypass vein grafts: results of a prospective randomized trial. J Vasc Surg 17: 382–398

Mills JL, Harris EJ, Taylor LM, Beckett WC, Porter JM (1990) The importance of routine surveillance of distal bypass grafts with duplex scanning: a study of 379 reversed vein grafts. J Vasc Surg 12: 379–389

Mills JL, Fujitani RM, Taylor SM (1993) The characteristics and anatomic distribution of lesions that cause reversed vein graft failure: a five-year prospective study. J Vasc Surg 17: 195–206

Sanchez LA, Gupta SK, Veith FJ, Goldsmith J, Lyon RT, Wengerter KR, Panetta TF, Marin ML, Cynamon J, Berdejo G, Sprayregen S, Bakal CW (1991) A ten-year experience with one hundred fifty failing or threatened vein and polytetrafluoroethylene arterial bypass grafts. J Vasc Surg 14: 729–738

Stierli P, Aeberhard P, Livers M (1992) The role of colour flow duplex screening in infra-inguinal vein grafts. Eur J Vasc Surg 6: 293–298

Wyatt MG, Muir RM, Tennant WG, Scott DJA, Horrocks M (1990) An objective comparison of four stress tests in the assessment of "at risk" femoro-distal grafts. J Cardiovasc Surg 31: 340–343

Wyatt MG, Muir RM, Tennant WG, Scott DJA, Baird RN, Horrocks M (1991) Impedance analysis to identify the at risk femorodistal graft. J Vasc Surg 13: 284–293

Subject Index

Printing: Saladruck, Berlin
Binding: Buchbinderei Lüderitz & Bauer, Berlin